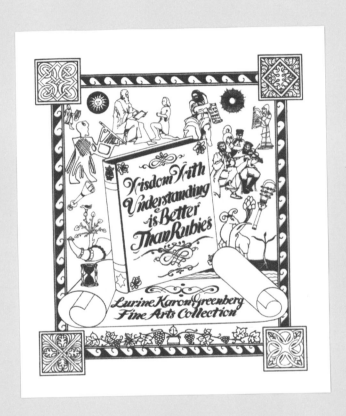

THE
ALZHEIMER'S
PREVENTION
COOKBOOK

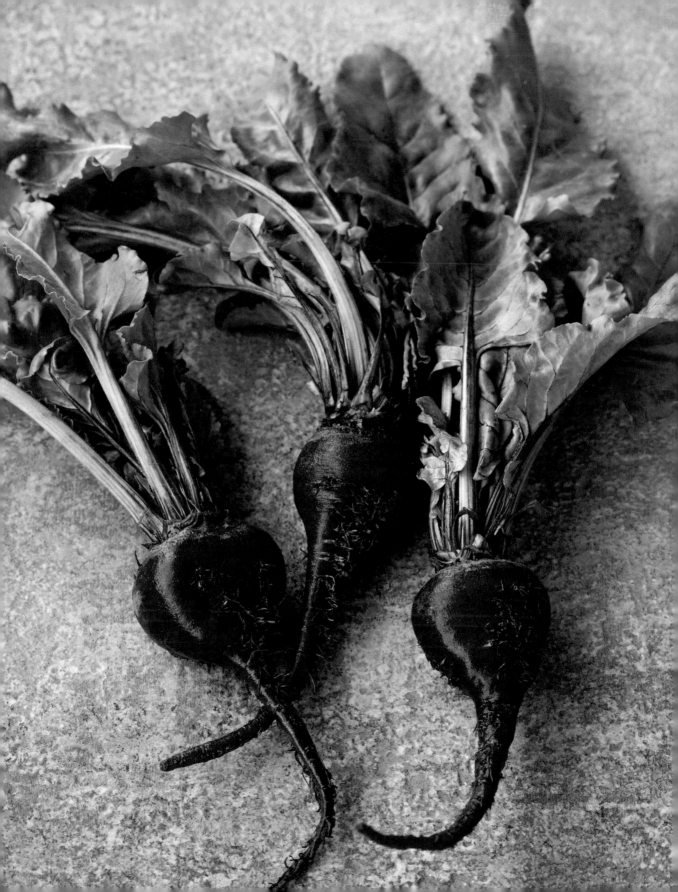

THE
ALZHEIMER'S
PREVENTION
COOKBOOK

Recipes to Boost Brain Health

Dr. Marwan Sabbagh and Beau MacMillan

PHOTOGRAPHY BY CAREN ALPERT

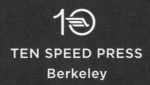

TEN SPEED PRESS
Berkeley

To my wife Ida and my two sons, Habib and Elias.

—MARWAN SABBAGH

Published in the United States by Ten Speed Press, an imprint of the
Crown Publishing Group, a division of Random House, Inc., New York.
www.crownpublishing.com
www.tenspeed.com

Ten Speed Press and the Ten Speed Press colophon are registered trademarks
of Random House, Inc.

Library of Congress Cataloging-in-Publication Data
is on file with the publisher.

All photographs are by Caren Alpert with the exception of the front cover
and page 139 by Leo Gong

ISBN 978-1-60774-247-0
eISBN 978-1-60774-248-7

Printed in China

Design by Chloe Rawlins
Food styling by Katie Christ
Prop styling by Carol Hacker

10 9 8 7 6 5 4 3 2 1

First Edition

Contents

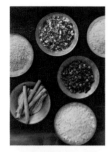
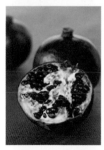
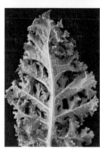

Acknowledgments

MARWAN:

This book would not be possible without the efforts of many people whose patience, passion, and dedication made my ideas come to life here. First, I want to thank my coauthor Beau MacMillan, who jumped into the project on faith. His enthusiasm has been inspiring. Next, I wish to thank Kari Stuart from International Creative Management who facilitated the book production and arrangement with Ten Speed. I want to thank the publication team at Ten Speed, particularly Sara Golski for her patience and skilled leadership in guiding Chef Beau and me through the process. This book is greatly enhanced in terms of content, language, and appeal because of the efforts of writer Laura Moser and photographer Caren Alpert. Both understood the project concept from the beginning and were able to bring the content to life in a wonderful and vibrant manner.

I also want to thank my family. My wife, Ida, and my sons, Habib and Elias, were patient with the all-consuming efforts that go into these book projects. I want to thank my dear friends Pat and Duffy McMahon for lending a kind and thoughtful ear to the project and then introducing me to Chef Beau. I want to acknowledge my assistant Myste Havens who set up countless conference calls for this project. Finally, I want to acknowledge my colleagues in the Arizona Alzheimer's Consortium and the Banner Sun Health Research Institute who stimulate my passion for Alzheimer's prevention and treatment, and most importantly, my patients, who every day make me understand why I do what I do.

BEAU:

I would like to extend my sincerest appreciation to Marwan for inviting me to take part in this amazing book. It has been an honor to work with him, and I am thankful for this opportunity and for everything I have learned from him along the way. I would also like to thank my sous chef, Russell LaCasce, for all of his support and devotion in helping compile these recipes. I am grateful to have had such a wonderful team at Sanctuary, who assisted me during throughout this process. Finally, I could not have imagined some of these recipes without the inspiration of fresh produce from Delightful Quality Produce. I am truly thankful to have had such tremendous support from everyone involved in making this book happen.

Introduction:
Preventing Alzheimer's Disease
with Nutrition

If you've picked up this book, it's probably because you've witnessed the ravages of Alzheimer's disease on someone you love—perhaps your mother or father, or even your sister or brother—and you fear the day when you might find yourself in the same position.

You're not alone. Alzheimer's ranks among the greatest health-care crises of the twenty-first century, and the numbers become even more dire with every passing year. According to the Alzheimer's Association, there are currently 5.4 million people diagnosed with Alzheimer's disease in the United States alone and up to 27 million affected people worldwide. In the States, they're nurtured by 14.9 million unpaid caregivers. According to the Alzheimer's Association, these nearly 15 million Alzheimer's and dementia caregivers provide 17 billion hours of unpaid care valued at $202 billion annually. Because of the toll this takes on their own health, these caregivers had $7.9 billion in additional health-care costs in 2010. Many of these caregivers are simultaneously parenting healthy young family members, a distinction that's earned them the unenviable label of the "sandwich" generation. As they struggle to care for both younger and older loved ones, they often fail to take care of their own health in the process—a perfectly understandable, but potentially hazardous, oversight. As a result, many of them suffer from higher rates of health problems, particularly depression.

With the rapidly aging baby boomer population, Alzheimer's disease—currently the sixth leading cause of death in the United States—will continue to affect more and more of us. Some estimate that one in eight baby boomers could develop Alzheimer's. In the first six years of this century, while deaths from stroke, prostate cancer, breast cancer, heart disease, and HIV fell, Alzheimer's disease deaths increased by a shocking 66 percent. Approximately one in every *ten* Americans over the age of sixty-five now suffers from Alzheimer's, and every year, an estimated 100,000 people die from the disease.

Alzheimer's affects so many of us: we either have a loved one who suffers from it, or know someone whose life has been drastically altered by caring for a relative or friend with the disease. The total cost of caring for Alzheimer's patients in 2011 was a staggering $183 billion, an $11 billion increase over the preceding year. This figure will continue to rise if we don't take immediate steps to protect the long-term health of our brains.

There is, of course, no known cure for Alzheimer's disease to date. Once a patient has been diagnosed with Alzheimer's (and this seldom happens before the disease has progressed far beyond the mildest stages), doctors can do little to stop the devastation. Treatment options are limited at this point, and while medications can improve symptoms, they have no real effect on the disease itself.

But the news isn't all grim. I'm here to tell you that there are easy, concrete steps every single one of us can take to avoid adding to the ranks of Alzheimer's sufferers and becoming just another sobering statistic. Even taking risk factors into account, we can fight to delay the onset of Alzheimer's altogether—and one of the most effective ways of doing this is to retool our diets. That's right. Eating better might help your brain work better and ultimately might stave off Alzheimer's.

Sound too good to be true? Well, a number of recent large, population-based studies have provided strong evidence linking a higher dietary intake of specific foods—those rich in the B-complex vitamins (especially B_6, B_{12}, and folates), anti-oxidants, anti-inflammatories, and unsaturated fatty acids—to a lower risk of developing Alzheimer's. Common foods, many of which you already have in your kitchen, can be your frontline weapons in the battle against dementia and cognitive decline. And if those benefits weren't enough to convince you, you'll also be combating obesity, cancer, heart disease, and a range of other ailments, some of which have been directly linked to Alzheimer's.

The inspiration behind this book is simple: With knowledge comes power. That is, with knowledge of current scientific findings, we gain the power to make potentially life-altering changes. And it is only after understanding this science—such as the damage free radicals do to the brain and body, and the link between the degenerative process of Alzheimer's and that of diabetes—that you will feel empowered to safeguard the health of your brain. This book is meant to empower you to take concrete steps toward reducing your risk of developing Alzheimer's. Since changes in the brain start decades before onset of symptoms, any modification you make now may reap huge rewards in future years.

I'm not saying acquiring this knowledge is a simple process, not at all—especially when there's still so much we don't know and the information changes so rapidly. We're bombarded daily with new and often contradictory information, and the constant updates can be confusing even to those of us who study Alzheimer's disease for a living. New studies seem to come out every day of the week, and the recommendations of one don't always line up with those in another. But while we are still a long way from conclusively understanding the interaction between environment and genetics that ultimately leads to the brain changes associated with Alzheimer's, we do have a good deal of useful, and potentially lifesaving, information at our disposal already. In fact, nutritional science research has identified trends in food consumption that appear to lead to lower rates of Alzheimer's and cognitive decline. That's the information we hope to put at your fingertips in *The Alzheimer's Prevention Cookbook*.

As a practicing medical doctor, geriatric neurologist, dementia specialist, and the director of research at a major teaching and learning institution, I'm engaged in investigations that make headline news. My colleagues and I have spent decades working to uncover the cause, treatment, prevention, and cure of Alzheimer's disease. Having led or participated in dozens of clinical trials and clinical research studies in Alzheimer's disease and other brain degenerative and medical conditions, I know exactly how overwhelming all the competing facts and figures out there can be. And that's another big reason I've written this book: to distill all the current research on how diet can alter your risk of developing Alzheimer's into straightforward language everyone can understand.

As a medical doctor, I'm daily confronted with the tragedy and devastation of Alzheimer's disease in the patients, and the fear and dread in the family members who take care of them. People—especially these legions of Alzheimer's caregivers—always ask what they can do to prevent getting the disease themselves. I tried to address that question in my first book, *The Alzheimer's Answer: Reduce Your Risk and Keep Your Brain Healthy*, which covered many aspects of Alzheimer's risk reduction but only touched on the all-important subject of diet.

Doctors and researchers have long advocated prescriptive diets for many conditions including heart disease, high cholesterol, high blood pressure, diabetes, and cancer. So why not Alzheimer's? Since we all must eat to stay alive, I wanted to write a book that focused on how diet affects Alzheimer's for better or worse, and how constructive changes in how and what we eat can have long-term benefits on our brains and bodies. The science of the brain continues to advance, and the more we learn about how our brains work, the more convinced we are that food can help us in the fight against Alzheimer's and dementia.

While there are still tremendous gaps in our knowledge, I'll start by focusing on what we *do* know. For example: We know that people with diets that are high in saturated fats and low in antioxidants and vitamins have higher rates of Alzheimer's disease. We know that obesity, diabetes, and other diet-related inflammatory conditions often correspond with, contribute to, or predate Alzheimer's diagnoses. We know that, even if you have a genetic predisposition to Alzheimer's, you could significantly delay the onset of symptoms for many years by adopting preventive strategies like dietary modification in your thirties through sixties.

And even a short delay would reap huge rewards for the entire US health-care system: if we could somehow manage to delay symptoms by even a year, we could bring down the prevalence of Alzheimer's by 5 percent by the year 2030. If, on the other hand, we sit back and do nothing to stop the rising tide of diagnoses, an estimated 14 to 16 million Americans will have Alzheimer's by 2050. In fact, some advocates and health economists predict that Alzheimer's could cost society $1 trillion dollars by midcentury if left unchecked. While researchers have long focused on developing innovative treatments for Alzheimer's once symptoms have manifested, a growing consensus maintains that preventing Alzheimer's is far preferable to treating it. That's why we've started paying so much attention to how our diets affect our brains: diet remains one of the easiest lifestyle factors to modify, and anyone can start making these changes right away.

There are, of course, caveats, and fairly large ones at that. For one thing, prevention is much harder to quantify than a cure—and the pharmaceutical industry is much more successful in treating symptoms than erasing the underlying disease.

While we could be waiting decades for an Alzheimer's cure, leading scientists now believe that we might be able to suppress, or delay the onset of, the awful illness. We're currently investigating a variety of dementia-fighting devices, including exercise, vitamins and supplements, hormone therapy, anti-inflammatory medications, cholesterol-lowering drugs, and—you guessed it—diet.

We had two primary motivations for writing a book about this last, and most promising, avenue of Alzheimer's prevention: (1) because a wide range of studies have already shown real brain-protective benefits of certain foods, and (2) because unlike hormone treatments and cholesterol drugs, good nutrition is available to everyone at minimal expense—and with no negative side effects.

I am not claiming that Alzheimer's is entirely preventable; it isn't. Certain risk factors—genetics, age, and gender—are unalterable for the foreseeable future. And we just don't know if even the healthiest of diets can altogether overcome a genetic predisposition to Alzheimer's. But that does not mean that developing Alzheimer's is inevitable, or that there's absolutely nothing we can do in the face of genetics.

While the genetic factors of Alzheimer's disease certainly shouldn't be ignored, there are many nongenetic causes as well, and these are the ones that deserve our attention—and intervention. Unhealthy dietary choices can lead to obesity and diabetes, which are in turn linked to Alzheimer's; healthy dietary choices can benefit both our brains and our waistlines.

So even if there's still a tremendous amount we've yet to learn about this incredibly complex disease, why not make the most of the ample knowledge that we already possess? Can we really afford to wait for every scientific fact and discovery to be proven beyond a shadow of a doubt? Absolute certainty might take decades. With Alzheimer's rates spiraling upward at such out-of-control rates, can we really afford to adopt a passive approach? Why not take charge of our health proactively? That's the core philosophy behind *The Alzheimer's Prevention Cookbook*.

So yes, there *is* an alternative to waiting passively for a cure for Alzheimer's—or to waiting for Alzheimer's to set in. We've written this book to give you the culinary road map you need to make Alzheimer's prevention an achievable goal. Consider our plan a science-to-table-to-brain-health protocol (our spinoff of the farm-to-table concept). It's delicious, simple, fun, and extremely affordable (especially when compared to the estimated $30,000 to $70,000 spent annually treating each and every Alzheimer's sufferer in the United States).

And the lessons and recipes in this book won't just help you fight Alzheimer's. The potential upside is that adhering to the recommendations of the book may improve your cardiovascular and overall health as well, by trimming your waistline, improving your energy level, and reducing your susceptibility to other inflammatory diseases. By learning how to cook and eat smarter, you won't just be protecting your brain, but your whole body. And you can rest assured that your taste buds won't suffer in the process, either. In fact, they very well may thank you.

Much of our dietary plan depends on everyday fruits, vegetables, spices, and proteins, including pomegranates, leafy greens, cinnamon and other spices like turmeric, fish, and chicken. We borrow some of the healthiest and most delicious dietary tricks from all over the world, everywhere from the Mediterranean to South Asia, offering simple, delicious recipes that bring disease-prevention science right to your table.

And once again, it all starts with arming you with the right information. For instance, did you know that eating just three fish meals each week can reduce the risk of Alzheimer's disease by 40 to 60 percent, or that a single teaspoon of cinnamon provides more than the recommended daily dose of antioxidants, those free-radical-scrubbing powerhouses that directly combat the effects of aging? What about the fact that India has the lowest incidence of Alzheimer's disease in the world, and that scientists attribute this amazing statistic to South Asians' fondness for the spice turmeric? And if you knew that a half a teaspoon of cloves contains *double* the antioxidants you're supposed to get in a day, you'd surely eschew chocolate-chip cookies in favor of the humble ginger snap.

Through the magical talents of Chef Beau MacMillan, executive chef of Sanctuary on Camelback Mountain and its signature restaurant, the recipes in *The Alzheimer's Prevention Cookbook* transform turmeric, cinnamon, cloves, and a host of other proven protective ingredients into culinary friends as trusted as salt and pepper. But despite the inclusion of some standard Indian spices, this is not a book of vindaloos and heavy curries. All of the food in this book—from power bars and energy shakes to stews and simple salads—is tailored to the American palate. Chef MacMillan, who has cohosted the Food Network's hit series *Worst Cooks in America* and currently appears on their shows *The Best Thing I Ever Ate* and *Chopped: All-Stars*, knows all about making familiar food that's as nourishing as it is delicious. Chef Beau and I discussed at length which ingredients most help in the fight against Alzheimer's, and he brilliantly incorporated those ingredients into an array of healthful and delicious meals.

The Alzheimer's Prevention Cookbook is about making doable, scientifically based changes to our diets. Our recipes allow every reader—whether an experienced cook or a complete kitchen novice—to choose from daily prescriptive menus that include delicious recipes such as protein-packed Gingered Spinach, Chicken, and Sun-Dried Tomato Omelet (page 114), which provides a low-saturated-fat breakfast alternative; or Spiced Dried-Fruit Compote (page 214), which fulfills the daily requirements of antioxidants; Wild Rice with Root Vegetables (page 200), a quick, delicious dinner that shows just how easy it is to embrace the Mediterranean diet at home; Lamb Stew with Fragrant Spices (page 182), which allows the uninitiated to use turmeric in a standard American recipe; and our signature turmeric-accented Brain-Boosting Broth (page 130), which can form the base of virtually all soups.

So forget the food pyramid. Forget points, calories, and carbs versus proteins. Our philosophy is simple: feed your head first, and good health will follow. Our diet will revolutionize the way you eat. Instead of picking your way around the prescribed five servings a day of this and that, or counting calories, or solely watching carbohydrates, you'll strive to hit as near as possible a prescriptive daily dose of the foods that are believed to prevent Alzheimer's disease. In the process, you'll reduce your susceptibility to other inflammatory illnesses as well, including heart disease, cancer, and diabetes.

We call it "eating from the top down," a new and empowering way to think about food. Feeding your brain nourishes the body, protects your mind, and will forever improve your family's future health. So whether you're taking care of an aging parent or a houseful of young children—or just trying to take care of yourself—*The Alzheimer's Prevention Cookbook* will equip you to extend the healthy functioning of your brain and help you to feel great in the process.

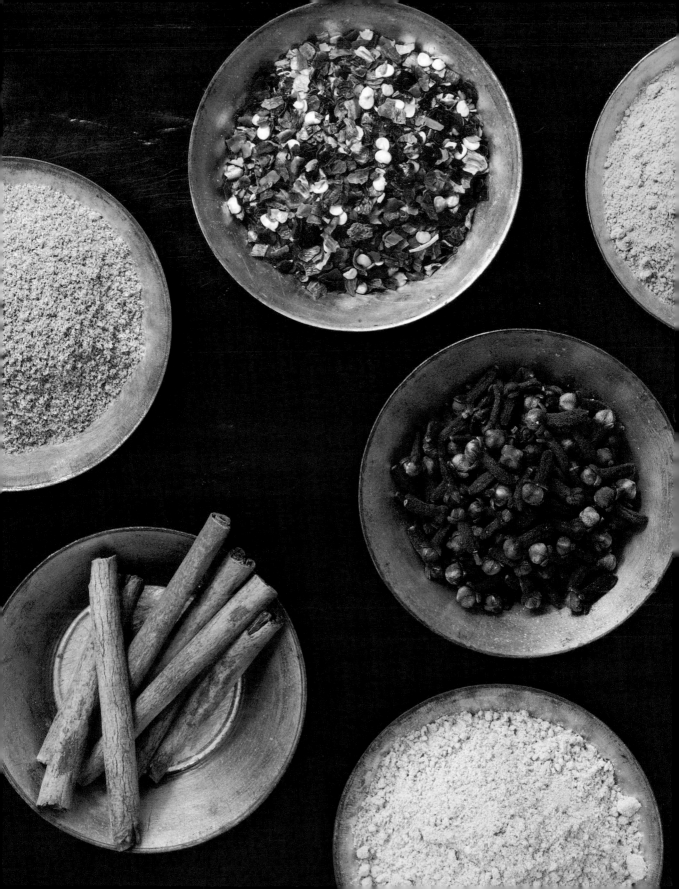

PART 1

THE SCIENCE OF ALZHEIMER'S DISEASE

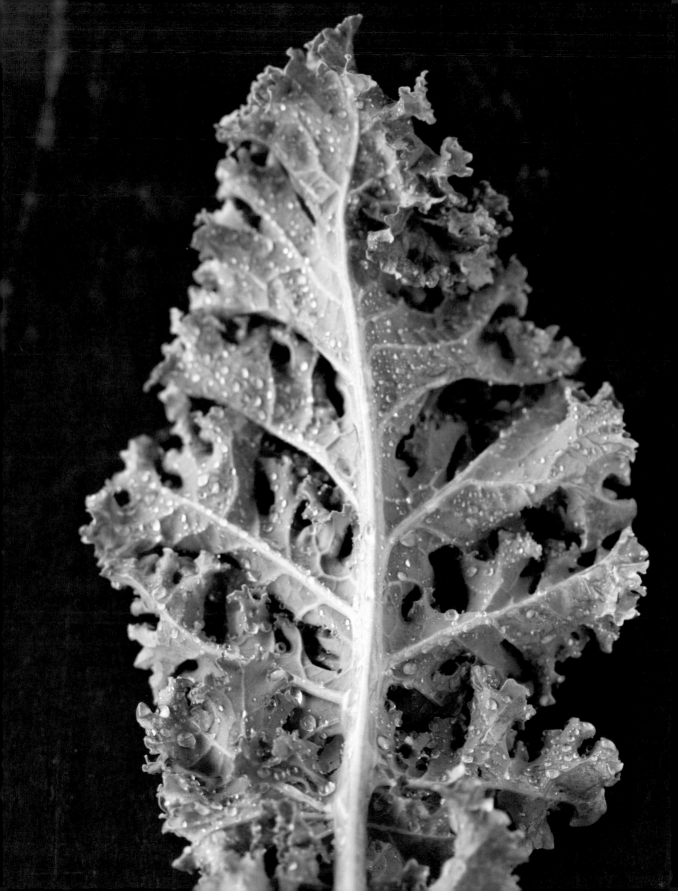

CHAPTER 1

What Is Alzheimer's Disease?

To understand how the food you eat can affect the future health of your brain, you first need a broad understanding of what Alzheimer's disease does to your brain. *Alzheimer's* is a degenerative progressive brain disease that impairs memory, language, thought, judgment, and behavior. It accounts for roughly half to two-thirds of cases of dementia, which is a category of disease just like cancer or heart disease. (*Dementia* refers to a condition where cognitive or memory impairment is severe enough to affect daily life; it does not by definition identify the underlying cause.) As Alzheimer's progresses, the cognitive decline that characterizes this disease slowly robs sufferers of their faculties and their ability to manage their personal habits and eventually other aspects of their health. Alzheimer's disease leads to death anywhere from three to twenty years after the onset of symptoms.

This paragraph contains a lot of scientific terminology, but please don't let it scare you. I'll define the terms and help you understand the role they play in Alzheimer's. Though scientists have been studying it for a little over a century, we still have a long way to go in understanding and treating Alzheimer's disease, which, as I've said, has no known cure, and none projected for the foreseeable future. While we have known for almost a century that Alzheimer's brains had distinctive features, including senile plaques, neurofibrillary tangles, and atrophy, it wasn't until 1984, almost eighty years after Dr. Alois Alzheimer first described the disease that would eventually take his name, that two researchers identified a protein composed of amyloid beta peptide, which is also called senile plaque.

Studying this amyloid plaque—the mechanisms by which the brain produces it, and the destruction it wreaks within the brain—has been the foundation of a good deal of Alzheimer's research ever since. Scientists have subsequently identified other features of the Alzheimer's-affected brain, including atrophy (shrinkage), loss of brain cells, loss of nerve connections, an accumulation of proteins known as *neurofibrillary tangles*, impairment of signaling within brain cells because they get jumbled up with these neurofibrillary tangles, loss of brain chemicals called *neurotransmitters* that send

PLAQUE AND THE BRAIN

Proteins are one of the principal building blocks of the human body. They're essential for the structure and function of all organs from skin and bones to the brain. And while they're essential for survival, there are also many degenerative conditions where proteins abnormally accumulate when they should not, including Alzheimer's, Huntington's, and Parkinson's. In these cases, the proteins might be a byproduct of normal or abnormal biochemical processes, or they might be overproduced, or they might not be cleared properly. In the case of Alzheimer's disease, amyloid plaque starts accumulating in the brain. This plaque is made up of cellular waste that has accumulated immediately outside the ends of cells. This waste is made up of proteins called amyloid and inflammatory molecules called cytokines, as well as of other components of cellular breakdown. In other words, the plaque is made of all the debris from dying or dead cells. At the heart of the plaque is a protein called amyloid, which is a byproduct of protein processing.

Normal amyloid is a protein molecule composed of forty amino acids (building blocks of proteins) aligned in a specific sequence. This molecule is generally cleared from the brain in much the same way that all cell waste is cleared away. Abnormal amyloid, called beta-amyloid protein, is composed of forty-two amino acids. It's very sticky and clumps together like lint, and once it does so, it is not easily removed or dissolved. As the plaques accumulate in the brain, they interfere with the normal processing of brain cells.

signals from one part of the brain to the other, loss of cellular self-maintenance abilities, and persistent inflammation.

Alzheimer's is a progressive disease, characterized by an inexorable march from mild to moderate to advanced dementia. It begins to surface in a transitional phase known as mild cognitive impairment, which I liken to the chest pain before the heart attack, or the mole before the melanoma. *Mild cognitive impairment*—a subtle condition characterized by selective memory loss that is apparent to the sufferer and to family and friends while not severe enough to affect the ability to complete tasks in a significant way—is of great interest to Alzheimer's researchers because we believe that at this stage there might still be a window of opportunity to delay, or even slow altogether, the progression to Alzheimer's. That said, many scientists, researchers, and medical doctors believe it may be too late to treat Alzheimer's at this stage. It's far preferable to prevent the disease even before the mild cognitive impairment state begins. That's why many of us place so much emphasis on prevention strategies, including diet, the overriding subject of this book.

I can't state this often enough: Stopping the clock on Alzheimer's before the fact is of crucial importance because, once a patient has been diagnosed, we're more or less unable to reverse the ravages to the brain. We cannot turn back the clock on memory loss once it's underway; we can do little more than stand by as the symptoms go from bad to worse.

The Progression of Alzheimer's: The Three Stages

Alzheimer's is a disease in three main stages, and the typical course can run anywhere from three to twenty years, with an average duration of about eight to ten years from the onset of memory loss to death. Once fully symptomatic Alzheimer's begins, each stage lasts between three and four years on average.

Most Alzheimer's diagnoses occur once a person is fully symptomatic, often in the moderate stage of the disease. Though many people seek care when their symptoms are still in the mild stage, far too many doctors dismiss their concerns as old age or some other malady.

Early onset Alzheimer's, or Alzheimer's that surfaces when the patient is sixty years old or younger, is quite rare, and most cases are associated with a genetic form of the disease and a strong family history. With early onset Alzheimer's, the symptoms seem to progress unabated despite medications, and it's still unclear whether prevention strategies would have any impact.

EARLY STAGE

In the early stage of Alzheimer's—which, like mild cognitive impairment, is often mistaken for normal aging—patients have trouble recalling new information and remembering words. People with mild Alzheimer's can have symptoms for three to five years. They tend to repeat themselves; forget appointments, phone calls, and conversations; and frequently get lost. They frequently misplace objects, have trouble driving, and exhibit signs of depression and anxiety. What distinguishes early stage Alzheimer's from mild cognitive impairment is when the memory impairment starts to affect daily life such as managing finances, cooking, and housekeeping. For example, say your mother was always in charge of cooking Thanksgiving dinner. Now that she's developing Alzheimer's, she can no longer remember which ingredients to buy or how to assemble them. Unless these mistakes are glaringly obvious or family members are paying close attention, many Alzheimer's sufferers can pass through this early phase without getting the medical attention they need.

INTERMEDIATE STAGE

In the intermediate stage, known as moderate Alzheimer's, patients have trouble remembering events in the distant past and confuse the past with the future. Their language skills regress to the point that they substitute words and lose their ability to identify objects or family members by name. At this stage, they also have trouble following conversations, and they often get lost. They have trouble recognizing people, even their relatives; become agitated or paranoid; and may develop delusions. They tend to get increasingly confused as the day progresses, a process that's known as "sundowning." By this stage, the impact on daily living is pervasive, and they can no longer live alone safely nor manage their affairs. The symptoms of anxiety, agitation, and depression worsen; they lose interest in favorite activities; and their sleep is often disturbed. This stage puts a lot of burden on family members because of the behavioral and sleep disturbances.

LATE STAGE

At the final, most heartbreaking stage of Alzheimer's, most patients are completely dependent on others for survival. Their memories, both short and long term, are severely impaired, and they often fail to recognize their loved ones or remember large chunks of their lives. Their speech suffers, often to the point of incomprehensibility, and they experience extreme agitation that can manifest itself in physical violence. They no longer understand that anything is wrong with them, and they often lose control of their bladder and bowels. Their movements become increasingly stiff; they lose the ability to walk or even sit upright; and they often forget to eat, or even to chew and swallow food already placed in their mouths. Some doctors claim that Alzheimer's disease does not cause death, but it clearly contributes to death as it robs patients of their basic abilities.

―――――――――――――

It's important to recognize that these devastating symptoms differ markedly from the normal aging process. Not all dementia is Alzheimer's—by no means. We all become more forgetful as we age, but forgetting where you left your keys is not the same thing as failing to recognize your husband of forty years. It bears repeating that *Alzheimer's is not just old age*: it can strike some people in their forties and fifties, while sparing others of far more advanced years. By far the best protocol is to take charge of your health now, and reap the benefits for the rest of your life.

Risk Factors

There are clearly identifiable risk factors for developing Alzheimer's. Some of these may be modifiable insofar as aggressive treatment can help minimize their impact on overall health; other risk factors are not modifiable. Recognizing the risks is the first step toward attempting to change their outcomes.

Unmodifiable Risk Factors

An *unmodifiable risk factor* is one that we cannot alter. These include our age, our gender, our family history, and, by extension, our genetic risk factors. Understanding that we cannot modify these risk factors puts the emphasis on offsetting their impact and focusing on strategies to promote brain health and taking steps as early as possible to engage in preventive strategies such as dietary modification. While having these factors is, of course, scary, we can minimize their impact by tackling them head on.

There are ways to identify one's risk. One option is the apolipoprotein E genotype blood test, but I only recommend that to patients who are already experiencing symptoms, as a positive result on a nonsymptomatic person can lead to long-term loss of insurance coverage. More often when I see a patient with a memory complaint, I add up their individual risk factors to determine if they are in a high-risk group or a low-risk group. In so doing, I can determine how aggressively I should treat their complaints.

AGE

Age is the most obvious risk factor for Alzheimer's: the longer you live, the higher your risk. At age sixty-five, 5 percent of people in the U.S. have Alzheimer's, and that risk roughly doubles every five years thereafter. Some experts estimate that by age eighty-five, as much as half the population might have Alzheimer's.

GENETIC INFLUENCES

While we don't fully understand how genetics affects Alzheimer's, we do know that it has a genetic component. More than 95 percent of all Alzheimer's cases are considered *multifactorial*, meaning they can be attributed to multiple causes, but the presence of three particular genes—amyloid precursor protein, presenilin I, and presenilin II—has been associated with a higher risk of developing the disease, especially in the case of early onset Alzheimer's. Family history is also a factor, and people whose relatives (especially first-degree relatives) suffer from the disease are about twice as likely to get the disease as nonrelatives, though we've yet to work out exactly why this is the case.

APOLIPOPROTEIN E GENOTYPE

The apolipoprotein E genotype, which refers to the specific genetic composition of a cell, organism, or individual, can be determined by a blood test that capable of identifying one of the most powerful Alzheimer's risk factors. This test simply tells which of three *apolipoproteins*, or blood proteins that carry fat and cholesterol in the blood to and from the liver, we have in our blood: APOE ε2, APOE ε3, and APOE ε4.

Research indicates that the rare APOE ε2 genotype might provide some protection against Alzheimer's. APOE ε3, the most common genotype, is neutral in terms of Alzheimer's risk. The APOE ε4 genotype, however, is found in about half the people with Alzheimer's disease. Like all blood types, APOE ε4 is inherited from both parents, and people who have two copies of APOE ε4 are *eighteen times* likelier than the general population to develop Alzheimer's, whereas people with only one copy of the APOE ε4 have a risk three to four times greater than for the general population.

FEMALE GENDER

We also know that more women than men develop Alzheimer's; as many as two to three times more women are affected. Again, we haven't yet isolated the reason for this discrepancy: it could have something to do with estrogen levels, since studies of brains of women who had died with Alzheimer's showed they had less estrogen than other women's brains.

Modifiable Risk Factors

And now for the risk factors that we have at least partial control over, many of which, you'll see, are directly related to cardiovascular health and weight. We've seen time and again that excess weight and the health conditions that go with it, like diabetes and high cholesterol, seem to accelerate Alzheimer's disease changes in the brain. The following have all been linked to Alzheimer's:

- Hypertension (high blood pressure)

- Elevated cholesterol

- Diabetes-elevated insulin levels (and metabolic syndrome)

- Heart disease and high homocysteine levels

- Cerebrovascular disease (strokes and transient ischemic attacks)

- Head injury

- Deficiency of folic acid (vitamin B9)

- Obesity, especially during midlife

Treatment of Alzheimer's

At the current time, as I've mentioned before, there is no known cure for Alzheimer's disease, though we've made some strides in treating it. Goals for Alzheimer's disease include improving memory, improving behavioral symptoms, preserving function (meaning present abilities), and slowing the progression of the disease and the decline of the patient.

The medications currently available have a modest but definite effect on Alzheimer's. They can improve such qualities as alertness, concentration, memory, and recall. Treatment goals also depend on the stage of disease. For early stage, the primary goal is to preserve mental functions. If, for example, people have stopped driving but can

EXERCISE AND ALZHEIMER'S

Physical exercise is another proven Alzheimer's-prevention strategy, and not simply because it keeps the weight down. People who exercise with pre-Alzheimer's symptoms have shown 10 to 20 percent improvement on memory tests. (Even people who don't have Alzheimer's symptoms who went from sedentary to active lifestyles had scored 5 to 10 percent higher on these memory tests.) Researchers believe a protein called *brain-derived neurotropic factor*, or BDNF, is responsible for these changes. BDNF, which is stimulated by exercise, can have a healing effect on the brain.

As the *New York Times* recently reported, the benefits of exercise seem to be even more dramatic with carriers of the APOE ε4 gene, who are more predisposed to develop Alzheimer's: those who exercised regularly—defined as 150 minutes a week of aerobic exercise, which is the same standard applied to cardiovascular disease—had plaque accumulation similar to those who did not carry the APOE ε4, which suggests that exercise counteracts the genetic component of Alzheimer's.[1] So whether you carry the gene or not, a thirty-minute walk or jog five days a week can help safeguard your body and brain.

LIMBERING UP YOUR BRAIN

You can exercise your brain in other ways as well. Crossword puzzles, Sudoku, foreign language acquisition, and even board games can all help keep your brain supple and sharp, although we don't exactly know why. One complicating factor is what's known as a *proxy effect* in play, meaning a person who does Sudoku tends to be more active, engaged, and educated than one who does not, and it's hard to examine this activity in isolation. The *dose effect* is also a big question mark: does a person who does Sudoku for three hours a day benefit three times as much as a person who does it for only one? As in so many areas of brain research, the details are hard to drill down, but it is clear that these activities have a protective effect on our brains. Though like many brain-training programs, the positive effects might last only as long as people do the activities: the improvements might not stick.

still handle their finances, the treatment goal is not to relearn how to drive, but rather to maintain the ability to do finances. The medication donepezil (Aricept) has been shown to delay this type of functional decline.

For intermediate-stage disease, the goal is to avoid the "big three": falls, incontinence, and behavioral disturbances, which are the principal reasons why people with Alzheimer's are placed into long-term care. Drugs used at this stage include donepezil (Aricept), rivastigmine (Exelon), galantamine (Razadyne), and tacrine (Cognex), which are known as *cholineterase inhibitors* because they slow the breakdown of *acetylcholine*, the neurochemical in the brain that is responsible for memory. While they don't stop Alzheimer's, these cholineterase inhibitors may well slow down its progression.

The more advanced Alzheimer's becomes, the more difficult it is to treat. A newer drug like memantine (Namenda), which has been approved for the treatment of moderate to severe Alzheimer's disease, is an *NMDA receptor antagonist*, meaning it protects brain cells from becoming overexcited. This overexcitement is related to the overproduction of a brain chemical called *glutamate*. When there is an excess of glutamate, the brain cells take in too much calcium, causing them to die.

As you can see, all of these treatment goals are unequal to the ravages of Alzheimer's disease. A far, far healthier—and more effective—approach is to fight the symptoms before the fact with food. Treat your brain right while it's still healthy, and you'll extend the life of your mind and body for many years to come.

CHAPTER 2

Food versus Supplements

So why, you might be asking, is what I eat so important? Why can't I just swallow a few vitamins with my morning OJ and be done with it? Because food is by far a more effective and (not to mention) delicious medicine, with more proven, sustained benefits.

In recent years, the efficacy of vitamins and nutritional supplements has become a hot topic in the medical and mainstream press alike. Drugstores and supermarkets stock their shelves with whole alphabets of vitamins, and millions of these bottles find their way into the medicine cabinets of consumers desperate to believe that these magic capsules will fortify them against horrible diseases such as Alzheimer's and cancer.

We love taking our daily vitamins. Popping a pill (or three) every morning makes us feel as if we're taking a concrete step toward wellness without actually having to do the heavy lifting involved in overhauling our diets, lifestyle, or exercise habits.

Indeed, many of us believe in the positive benefits of vitamins even when no rigorous clinical or scientific studies exist to substantiate this belief. The vitamin industry rakes in $16 billion a year in the States alone, a figure that could top $1 trillion as more and more of us seek a shortcut to improved health.[1]

Should vitamins be the touchstone of Alzheimer's prevention? I wish I could just say yes and be done with it. But while scientists have studied many different vitamins with an eye toward preventing and treating Alzheimer's—particularly vitamin C, vitamin E, and the B vitamins—there's still a good deal we don't know about how exactly these and other supplements might contribute to cognitive health. We have, it seems, placed unrealistically high hopes in supplements. While they've been shown to benefit certain conditions—omega-3s can be effective in reducing cardiovascular risk, for example—we know less about how they affect overall health. We also have larger, more basic unanswered questions about how particular nutrients can alter the brain, and how these neural changes can subsequently affect intelligence, mood, and behavior.

Studying the relationship between nutrition and the brain is endlessly complicated for many reasons:

1. Poor nutrition and environmental factors are interconnected, so behavioral changes might not be due to poor nutrition only but also to other factors such as education or social or family problems.
2. Because it's difficult to alter only one substance in the human diet, it's difficult to determine how (or if) a particular vitamin or mineral affects behavior. For ethical reasons, we cannot conduct experiments that prohibit a person from eating a particular nutrient, so much of the data comes from animal experiments. Human studies are generally limited to examining the effects of famine and starvation on health.
3. We respond to different diets in different ways. We all need, and process, different nutrients differently.

But even without all these complexities, the main reason we know that eating the right foods is more effective than taking vitamins and supplements at delivering Alzheimer's-fighting benefits has to do with something known as the *blood–brain barrier*, which acts as the gatekeeper of substances between the brain and the rest of the body. The blood–brain barrier is like a wall between the bloodstream and neurons: it prevents certain substances from penetrating the brain, while encouraging the absorption of others.

How Do Nutrients Reach the Brain?

For nutrients to deliver any benefit to our brains, they have to get there first—and this process is by no means a straightforward one. Nutrients must overcome several challenges on the tricky pathway into our brains:

1. The nutrients must gain entry to our bodies, meaning we must first consume them.
2. Once in the stomach, they must survive an attack by acid that breaks some foods down.
3. Further along the digestive tract, they must be absorbed through the cells lining the intestine and transported through blood vessel walls into the bloodstream.
4. Traveling in the blood through the liver, nutrients need to avoid being metabolized (in other words, used as energy and destroyed). The fact that supplements and vitamins are broken down more readily has the potential to diminish their impact. In other cases, supplements are not digested thoroughly or at all, which means they can pass through the entire digestive track without being absorbed.
5. Once in the bloodstream, nutrients must cross small blood vessels into brain tissue, a process restricted by the blood–brain barrier.

What Does the Blood–Brain Barrier Do?

The blood–brain barrier is an extremely effective filter that protects the brain from many common bacterial infections, which means that infections of the brain are very rare. (But since antibodies and antibiotics are too large to cross the blood–brain barrier, infections of the brain that do occur are often very serious and difficult to treat.) For the same reason, it's also difficult to target drugs to reach the brain, since the blood–brain barrier keeps out both toxins and potentially therapeutic chemicals.

The blood–brain barrier becomes more permeable during injuries including stroke, head trauma, meningitis, encephalitis, and multiple sclerosis. In these circumstances, some antibiotics and other medication—substances ordinarily kept out of the blood–brain barrier—can cross into the brain. Viruses, too, can easily bypass the blood–brain barrier by attaching themselves to circulating immune cells.

But in healthy people, when the blood–brain barrier is functioning properly, food nutrients stand a much better chance of passing into the brain than supplements for the simple reason that the body has already done the job of breaking these nutrients down into smaller, easily transported molecules. Because supplements are frequently broken down during the digestion process, they may be altered and lose their intended effect. When supplements aren't broken down, their molecules often remain too large to complete the journey past the blood–brain barrier.

Should We Be Wary of Supplements?

In a word, yes: Supplements can be useful in—as their name suggests—*supplementing* a well-balanced diet, but they should never be used as *substitutes* for real food. Even in the cases where supplements do pass through the blood–brain barrier, we should never rely too much on nutrients in pill form, especially when it comes to the delicate chemistry of our brains.

These days, it can be hard to resist the lure of perfect health in a bottle. More and more companies are peddling herbal remedies, vitamin formulas, and "medical foods" like Axona and Cerefolin that promise to enhance the memory or to delay or prevent Alzheimer's disease and related disorders. But while some of these remedies may be valid candidates for treatments, the science remains, for the most part, sketchy at best.

We have legitimate concerns about using these supplements as an alternative or in addition to physician-prescribed therapy:

- **Effectiveness and safety are unknown.** Because the U.S. Food and Drug Administration (FDA) doesn't require the same rigorous scientific research for dietary supplements as for prescription drugs, most of what we know about supplements derives from testimonials and a relatively small body of peer-reviewed research. Another issue is that the FDA only requires that supplements meet a standard called GRAS (generally recognized as safe). There is no requirement that the ingredients listed need to be in the tablets or in the amounts listed, and the manufacturers don't even have to establish that the supplements work as stated.

- **Purity is unknown.** Again, because the FDA has no authority over supplement production, the manufacturer must develop and enforce its own guidelines for ensuring that its products are safe and contain the ingredients listed on the label in the specified amounts. As a result of this lax regulation, supplements can have some serious quality-control issues. More expensive doesn't necessarily mean higher quality, and buying a supplement from a major drugstore chain in no way guarantees its safety.

- **Bad reactions are not routinely monitored.** Supplement manufacturers aren't required to report consumers' problems with their products to the FDA, so we don't know all their potential side effects. (The agency does provide voluntary reporting channels for manufacturers, health-care professionals, and consumers, and will issue warnings about a product when there is cause for concern.) The FDA also does little to monitor the source of supplements, so we have no assurance that they're not tainted with heavy metals or toxins.

- **Supplements can have serious interactions with prescribed medications.** Since manufacturers aren't required to list potential drug interactions on the supplement labels, many people might not even know that they may be mixing incompatible substances. For example, the memory supplement ginkgo biloba interacts with the blood thinner warfarin (Coumadin) to cause the blood to become too thin, but you wouldn't know this from looking at the ginkgo biloba label. No one should take a supplement without first consulting a physician.

- **The consistency and concentration of supplement dosages can vary widely.** Because supplement companies aren't held to the same rigorous manufacturing standards as pharmaceutical companies or food manufacturers, the dosage might be vastly different from tablet to tablet and bottle to bottle: a 1,000 mcg (microgram) tablet of vitamin B12 might contain 100 mcg or 10,000 mcg.

We also have some questions about the efficacy of supplements. Supplements have varying amounts of *bioavailability*, which refers to the amount of nutrient absorbed, and the figure tends to be lower from supplements than from food. The industry average is 50 percent or less.

Another issue is that most supplements are extracted from food sources, which might have hidden nutritional benefits that don't translate into supplement form.

Many studies attempting to link certain nutrients with cognitive benefits have reached different conclusions when the nutrients have been ingested in supplement form rather than as an unprocessed food. Researchers believe that natural dietary sources might confer broad, wide-ranging health benefits whereas supplements might produce narrower, more selective benefits. For example, we presume that the benefit of eating fish comes from the fact that it is a good source of omega-3 fatty acids, but there might be other benefits to eating the whole fish that we haven't discovered yet. That's why we recommend getting your omega-3s from actual fish rather than relying wholly on supplements.

And before we can authoritatively single out certain nutrients for their brain-protecting properties, we need to learn more about the biological interaction between different nutrients. It could well be the interaction between nutrients that's responsible for many of the perceived health benefits, meaning the protection might come from a combination of many different nutrients rather than one in isolation.

Here's another reason we should focus on our diets rather than our vitamin cabinets: because the data supports it. Most of the evidence researchers have gathered on human nutrition uses surveys to estimate amounts of items consumed, and it's far easier to quantify dietary elements than supplement dosages. For example, while you can estimate a serving of fish, there are hundreds of different omega-3 supplements on the market, each containing different quantities of docosahexaenoic acid (DHA) and eicosapentaenoic acid (EPA). Or if, say, we were surveying orange consumption, we could quantify how many oranges a person eats every week. But if we attempted a similar estimate with vitamin C supplements, we'd find that people take different doses, ranging from 50 to 5000 mg a day, and that's without factoring in differences in quality from brand to brand. Vitamin C consumed in food sources adds another layer of complication.

Aside from these issues, food is the most natural source of nutrition, and a well-balanced diet has been shown to exert a protective benefit over time. We just don't have enough evidence to prove that supplements offer the same advantages. In fact, no studies have shown that supplements protect our health as effectively as diet, with the exception of omega-3s for cardiovascular disease and in cases of extreme nutritional deficiency syndromes (pellagra, scurvy, vitamin B_{12} deficiency).

Last but not least, the medical community and the FDA can't ever seem to agree on which supplements we should take and in what doses. That's mainly because the *recommended daily allowances* (RDA) guidelines set the minimum daily amounts of vitamins and minerals needed, but don't establish ideal daily quantities, to say nothing of how the levels of nutrients we take can address specific health conditions.

A final reason dietary protocols trump a supplement regimen every time is because we obtain most neurotransmitters—the brain chemicals that send signals from one part of the brain to the other—from the foods we consume. Certain foods contain *precursors* for neurotransmitters, most famously the tryptophan in eggs and turkey that helps make serotonin, which regulates our moods and helps us sleep. If a diet is deficient in these precursors, the balance of neurotransmitters becomes upset, and a number of mental and neurological issues can develop.

Here more than ever, supplements are no stand-in for proper nutrition. Because of the way we digest food and nutrients, the best source of neurotransmitter precursors is almost always food; supplements are *much* less reliable. As already described, the road from our mouths to our brain is long and winding. Since neurotransmitters are proteins, they won't be absorbed by the brain in the same form that we consume them. When neurotransmitters are embedded in food, the digestion process is more complex and the protein is more likely to be absorbed. By contrast, when we take neurotransmitters in supplement form, they might get broken down by our stomach acids before they come anywhere near our brains.

For example, taking the supplement choline to make the neurotransmitter acetylcholine doesn't benefit the brain because choline is digested in the stomach and never makes it across the blood–brain barrier. This is especially important for our purposes because acetylcholine is the neurotransmitter used for memory, and the one that's lost in Alzheimer's-afflicted brains. While it might sound like a great idea in theory, numerous studies have shown that ingesting acetylcholine precursors in supplement form doesn't improve cognition in Alzheimer's brains. Ingesting choline through food—it's found in egg yolks, liver, and soybeans—is a far better alternative. Choline is also found in whey powder, which you can add to everything from protein shakes to pancakes and muffins.

As always, the best way to get essential nutrients into our brain is through food, which is why we've written this book: to show you all the delicious ways that you can feed your brain the nutrients it needs to stay supple and sharp. Let's start with one of the most essential—and most readily available—brain-boosting nutrients we can increase in our diets: B-complex vitamins.

CHAPTER 3

Vitamin B and the Brain

For years now, we've known that B-complex vitamins have myriad health benefits, including a lowered risk of heart disease, diabetes, and anemia. B vitamins—a whole family of closely related vitamins that consists of vitamin B_1 (thiamin), B_3 (niacin), B_5 (pantothenic acid), B_6 (pyridoxine), B_9 (folic acid), and B_{12} (cyanocobolamin)—can also boost the digestive and immune systems, preserve the skin, and maybe even fight cancer.

More recently, scientists have begun to investigate the relationship between cognitive health and B vitamins. Recent epidemiologic data has shown that dietary sources of B vitamins, especially pyridoxine, folic acid, and B_{12}, can protect us against Alzheimer's and other forms of cognitive decline and dementia, with several studies demonstrating a link between cognitive decline in the elderly and low levels of these B-complex vitamins.

THE MOST IMPORTANT VITAMINS FOR BRAIN HEALTH

Remember, the three most important vitamins for brain health are B_6, B_9 (folic acid), and B_{12}.

As in so many areas of Alzheimer's research, we still have a lot to learn. While we've seen tangible evidence of their benefits time and again, we know very little about *why* B vitamins seem to do such a good job of protecting the brain. All we know is that a B12 deficiency can be a direct cause of dementia, and there's a consistent association between deficiencies in B-complex vitamins, or low levels of vitamin B in the blood, and an increased risk of Alzheimer's.

More generally, B-complex vitamins are essential for the nervous system to function. In contrast to many vitamins, B vitamins in supplement form have been shown to boost certain aspects of cognitive function. B vitamins are *water soluble*, meaning the body tends to eliminate them through urine. Because they're not stored in large amounts in the body, they're unlikely to reach toxic levels. And best of all, B vitamins are present in just about every natural food you can name. Most of us already get adequate levels of B vitamins in our diets, though less than we used to now that so many grains are processed and stripped of their natural nutrients. Some people, however, have trouble actually absorbing these vital nutrients in both dietary and supplement form, especially as they age. The only solution is to eat even *more* B-complex vitamins, thereby increasing the chances that adequate levels are absorbed by the stomach and small intestine. The older you get, the more B-complex vitamins you need to be eating.

B1, or **thiamin**, is directly involved in the brain's metabolic functions, and can help with reaction time and mental energy. A sudden drop in thiamin levels, most often caused by heavy alcohol consumption, can lead to confusion, vision problems, and difficulties with balance and walking. Acute thiamin deficiency as a result of frequent alcohol intoxication is called *Wernicke's encephalopathy*, a condition that's characterized by delirium, trouble walking, and impaired eye movements. When a thiamin deficiency becomes chronic, a type of dementia, called *Korsakoff dementia*, emerges. This type of dementia is characterized by an inability to plan and complete tasks, and short-term memory loss with confabulation (making things up to fill in memory gaps). Good food sources of thiamin include pork, oatmeal and other whole (as opposed to refined) grains, asparagus, romaine lettuce,

THIAMIN-RICH RECIPES

Roasted Eggplant Hummus (page 120)

Sautéed Mushrooms with Spinach and Black Vinegar (page 187)

Not-Your-Average Steel-Cut Oatmeal (page 104)

Banana, Granola, and Yogurt Parfaits (page 106)

mushrooms, spinach, black beans, green beans, pinto beans, lima beans, lentils, sunflower seeds, tuna, green peas, tomatoes, eggplant, and brussels sprouts.

B₃, or **niacin**, is important for glucose metabolism, and has been shown to increase blood flow and lower cholesterol. And while we've long known that severe niacin deficiency can cause dementia, researchers have recently begun to investigate whether dietary levels of niacin might also have some effect on age-related neurodegeneration or the development of Alzheimer's.[1] Increasing your dietary intake of niacin may protect you against Alzheimer's and age-related cognitive decline. It's fairly easy to get niacin in your diet: it's present in liver, chicken, beef, fish (tuna, salmon, halibut), mushrooms (particularly shiitake and crimini), cereal, seeds, peanuts, legumes, lamb, venison, avocados, and vegetables ranging from asparagus to leafy greens. Niacin is also synthesized from the neurotransmitter precursor tryptophan, which is found in meat, dairy, and eggs. However, the benefits of eating these foods—especially beef and full-fat dairy—might be offset by the harm they might cause in terms of increasing body weight, which, as we'll see, is a risk factor for Alzheimer's.

B₅, or **pantothenic acid**, is essential for the production of carbohydrates, fats, and proteins. In the brain, vitamin B₅ plays a role in the production of acetylcholine, a crucial neurotransmitter involved in learning and memory, and the one that is lost in Alzheimer's disease. You can get pantothenic acid in egg yolks, broccoli, liver, and brewer's yeast. Fish, shellfish, chicken, milk, yogurt, legumes, mushrooms, avocados, and sweet potatoes are also good sources. Whole grains also contain pantothenic acid, but the processing and refining of grains may result in a 35 to 75 percent loss of the nutrient. Freezing and canning foods can have a similar effect.

B₆, or **pyridoxine**, assists in the balancing of chemicals such as sodium and potassium. In the brain, pyridoxine is necessary to produce important neurotransmitters, including serotonin, dopamine, noradrenaline, and adrenaline. Dietary sources of B_6 include rice and wheat bran, dried herbs and spices, raw garlic, sunflower and sesame seeds, pistachios, hazelnuts, certain fish, bananas, salmon, turkey, chicken, potatoes, spinach, and vegetable juice.

B_9, or **folic acid (folate)**, is one of the few vitamins whose specific isolated total intake has been significantly associated with a lowered risk of Alzheimer's. Low folate levels are associated with poor cognitive function and dementia in the elderly, whereas the literature suggests that supplement-delivered folic acid may help protect against Alzheimer's.[2]

Folic acid deficiencies are rare in the United States today, a fact that is attributed to its nationwide supplementation in grain products. It's also easy to get folic acid as a single vitamin, in multivitamins, or in B-complex vitamins, and these supplements can be just as effective as dietary sources—a rare exception to the rule. But again, because you can't overdose on B vitamins, and because you need folates more than ever as you get older, you should make an effort to incorporate these brain-preserving nutrients into your diet as well. Good dietary sources of folates include asparagus, broccoli, lettuce, and cauliflower; leafy greens like spinach and kale; and legumes like lentils, peas, and beans. Corn, eggs, baked potatoes, and fruits like bananas, strawberries, and oranges also contain folate.

B_{12}, or **cyanocobolamin**, could be the single most important vitamin for neuronal health. It helps build the coating, or myelin sheaths, around nerve cells. Vitamin B_{12} deficiencies have been closely linked with spinal cord and nerve damage, memory loss, and dementia. Treatment with high-dose B vitamins has been shown to protect against heart attacks, strokes, and death. A population-based study published in *Stroke* in 2005 showed that people who took the highest dose of B_{12} were significantly less likely to suffer a stroke or heart attack. This study relied on B_{12} in supplement form

B_6-RICH RECIPES

Breakfast Fried Rice with Scrambled Eggs (page 111)

Green Tea–Pomegranate Smoothie (page 93)

Ahi Tuna on Rye with Spinach Pesto Yogurt (page 158)

Turkey on 9-Grain with Black Bean Salsa and Tarragon Yogurt (page 160)

Grilled Herbed Chicken Breasts with Sesame–Green Onion Rice and Bok Choy (page 176)

FOLATE-RICH RECIPES

Banana-Kale Wake-Up Smoothie (page 98)

Arctic Char with Grilled Red Onion (page 166)

Red Lentils with Kale and Miso (page 202)

Cannellini Beans with Parsnip and Celery Root (page 204)

B12-RICH RECIPES

Crab Salad with Saffron
(page 119)

Lamb Stew with Fragrant
Spices (page 182)

Braised Mussels with Garlic
and Chorizo (page 173)

VITAMIN B-BOOSTER RECIPES

These recipes contain a
range of different brain-protective B vitamins:

Avocado and Asian Pear
Smoothie with Ginger
(page 98)

Gingered Spinach, Chicken,
and Sun-Dried Tomato
Omelet (page 114)

Grilled Corn, Edamame, and
Tomato Salad (page 147)

because supplements, in this case, were easier to quantify, and foods high in B12 also happen to be high in saturated fats. That's because most dietary sources of B12 derive from animals: you can get it in liver (pâté and sausage included), shellfish (clams, oysters, and mussels have the highest content; crab and lobster are also a good source); fatty fish (and that includes caviar!); beef, lamb, and eggs. Most of these foods are good in moderation but not in excess, so be sure you're getting B12 in supplement form as well.

As the foods listed above indicate, B vitamins are everywhere, and it's not too difficult to fit more of them into your diet. You can get general B-complex vitamins in whole grains, potatoes, bananas, lentils, chile peppers, beans, nutritional yeast, brewer's yeast, and molasses.

As always, the key is to eat these foods regularly, since, as we'll see in chapter 7, a *composite diet*, meaning everything you eat over the course of a day from a variety of sources, provides the best defensive culinary action against Alzheimer's and other inflammatory diseases. Research also strongly suggests that it is a daily, long-term, dietary intake of high doses that have the greatest effect on our brains and bodies.

THE B-VITAMIN HALL OF FAME

While B vitamins are present in a huge range of foods, these foods contain the highest levels:

- Whole grains (as unprocessed as possible)
- Legumes like lentils and beans
- Bananas
- Leafy greens like spinach and kale

CHAPTER 4

Preventing Cell Damage with Antioxidants

*A*ntioxidants are substances that may protect cells from the damage caused by free radicals, which have been linked to environmental exposures like tobacco smoke and radiation. *Free radicals*—unstable molecules produced by various chemical reactions in the body—and other *reactive oxygen species* (chemically reactive species that contain oxygen, including superoxide, singlet oxygen, and hydrogen peroxide) can damage cells, and may play a role in heart disease, cancer, and other diseases. Free radicals also increase as we age, and our bodies become less capable of scavenging them and breaking them down.

While the human body does have a number of systems for eliminating free radicals and other byproducts of *oxidative stress* (a general term for the imbalance between the body's production of reactive oxygen species and its ability to detoxify these chemicals, discussed more fully later in this chapter) from the body, it is not 100 percent efficient. Oxidative stress refers to damage to our cells—and the organs and tissues composed of those cells—that results from our body's chemical reaction to the breakdown of oxygen inside our cells. If left unchecked, oxidative stress may lead to extreme cell damage and even cancer. By reducing oxidative stress and stabilizing the free radicals within our bodies, antioxidants may safeguard our cells from the level of damage that can lead to disease.

Examples of antioxidants include the following:

- Vitamin C

- Vitamin E

- Polyphenols

- Selenium

- Beta-carotene

Oxidative stress has been implicated in a range of serious health conditions, including atherosclerotic heart disease and cancer. And a growing body of evidence implicates such oxidative cellular damage in the brains of those with Alzheimer's disease as well.

Having extensively studied the role of antioxidants in preventing these and other diseases, researchers have concluded that antioxidants work in a number of ways: they may lessen oxidation by scavenging and inactivating free radicals, they may restore at least some normal functioning to tissues damaged by oxygen free radicals, or they may do a little bit of both.[1]

As with the saturated-fat studies, most evidence we have of antioxidants' protective effects comes from data gathered in animal research. These studies have shown that animals genetically engineered to get Alzheimer's disease who were fed high-antioxidant diets demonstrate superior memory (as measured by how well they learned how to navigate through mazes or remembered other conditioned tasks), reduced oxidative stress, and lower rates of cognitive decline than those fed lower amounts of antioxidants. But however encouraging these findings, reproducing these effects in humans has proven difficult.

Oxidative Stress

Wouldn't it be great if we could see oxidative stress like we see rust, another form of oxidation, on our cars? Unfortunately, the process of oxidative stress inside our bodies is far more complicated, and we can't replace parts of our body like we can a rusty fender.

As mentioned earlier, oxidative stress results from our body's chemical reaction to the breakdown of oxygen inside our cells.

Here's roughly how it works: We're all composed of chemicals, mostly water. The biochemical process is just like eating. We eat; we make and expend energy; we produce and expel waste. These are all normal chemical reactions that make the body run. In order to convert energy that we need to live, *mitochondria*—the "batteries" in cells that make them go—require oxygen. And, at the biochemical level, all of these chemical reactions have byproducts, such as carbon dioxide and water.

The purpose of our respiratory and circulatory systems is twofold: to deliver this oxygen to the tissues for use by mitochondria, and to eliminate carbon dioxide. But sometimes, eliminating the carbon dioxide isn't such a straightforward process. The byproducts of the chemical reactions that take place inside our bodies can have extra ions, or be difficult to eliminate from the system, or even be toxic. In the case of reactive oxygen species, these chemicals do great harm to the body.

I occasionally use a disgusting but effective analogy to help illustrate this process: Normal stool tends to be brown and firm. Abnormal stool might be green and loose. Free radicals and reactive oxygen species are, like the green stool, abnormal byproducts of a normal metabolic process. The free radicals produced by oxidation can start chain reactions, which—because they take place at the molecular level—can damage cells, tissue, and even DNA. This damage can greatly accelerate the aging process, since our cells must expend considerable energy attempting to heal and accelerate.

When an imbalance develops between what are known as *pro-oxidants* (which cause these abnormal oxygen byproducts to form and damage cells), and antioxidants (which scavenge these oxygen byproducts and protect the cells from damage), our cells undergo oxidative stress—a type of invisible rusting inside the body. And that's when things get messy.

Multiple studies suggest that oxidative stress is the leading cause of cardiovascular disease. It's also a big contributor to the aging process. Within brain cells, it's a suspected cause of all sorts of neurodegenerative diseases including Lou Gehrig's disease, Parkinson's disease, and Huntington's disease. And, most relevantly for our purposes, oxidative stress has been detected in brain, cerebrospinal fluid, blood, and urine of people with Alzheimer's.

So does oxidative stress cause Alzheimer's? We've yet to prove it, but we have identified an association between genetic and lifestyle-related risk factors for Alzheimer's disease and an increase in oxidative stress within the body. These findings suggest that oxidative stress is a factor early on in the development of Alzheimer's, which means that lowering our levels of oxidative stress might also lower our probability of developing Alzheimer's.

So what's the easiest and most efficient way to fight oxidative stress? Increase our intake of antioxidants.

Antioxidants in Supplement Form

Researchers are looking at the potential brain-boosting benefits of certain antioxidant supplements, particularly vitamins C and E. As always, the evidence seems to suggest that food is more reliable than supplements at getting nutrients into the diet.

VITAMIN C

Championed most famously by the Nobel Prize–winning chemist Linus Pauling, vitamin C is many people's go-to vitamin for warding off infections and maintaining general good health. Studies have demonstrated vitamin C's antioxidant, *antiatherogenic* (meaning it can prevent buildup of blockages in arteries), *anticarcinogenic* (meaning it can help fight cancer), antihistamine, antiviral, and antihypertensive properties. The FDA also recommends vitamin C for iron deficiencies. And since vitamin C is water soluble, we expel excess amounts in our urine before they become toxic to our systems (although too much can cause an upset stomach or diarrhea in some individuals). Vitamin C has been the subject of extensive investigations as it relates to cognitive aid and intelligence. A famous study reported in 1988 by David Benton and Gwilym Roberts of schoolchildren from kindergarten to college showed that students' IQ scores raised an average of nearly four points when their vitamin C intake was elevated by 50 percent through supplements.[2] Unfortunately, the connection between vitamin C intake and increased cognitive function has not been borne out across all studies.

VITAMIN E

Vitamin E has been consistently shown to have anti-Alzheimer's properties in cell cultures. It might even inhibit amyloid plaque formation and the neurotoxic effects of amyloid. (Amyloid is the building block of the plaque associated with Alzheimer's, and hundreds of studies have shown that amyloid can damage brain cells directly. That's why it's never desirable for amyloid to accumulate in the brain.) Not only that, but vitamin E also protected against reactive oxygen species and displayed anti-inflammatory properties.[3]

Studies in the 1990s suggested that high doses of vitamin E actually slowed down the progression of Alzheimer's, but studies ten years later failed to demonstrate any benefit in people with pre-Alzheimer's disease. And unlike vitamin C, there are risks in taking too much Vitamin E, so exercise caution if you're considering a vitamin E supplement, as high dosages might be harmful to the heart.

As this evidence proves, there's no magic bullet here: purified antioxidants in supplement form can't always deliver us the levels of nutrients we need. Unlike the dietary antioxidant studies, those of vitamin C and E supplements have so far shown negligible impact on participants' risk of developing Alzheimer's.[4]

Most of the current evidence suggests that gradual, sustained modifications to your diet will have a far greater impact on your brain health—and in the case of vitamin E, be much safer—than short-term, concentrated doses of supplements. Several large population-based surveys have found that a high dietary intake of antioxidant nutrients may be associated with a reduced risk of Alzheimer's and slower cognitive decline. So if you have a choice between a handful of vitamin E–rich sunflower seeds and a capsule of vitamin E, reach for the seeds every time.

Getting Antioxidants into Your Diet

So if supplements don't provide adequate protection, what's the best way to increase your intake of antioxidants? You guessed it: through a steady, diet-based source. And while you can all too easily overdose on supplements, there's no such thing as *eating* too many antioxidants. On the contrary, by choosing the right foods, you can lower your oxidative stress and possibly reduce your risk of developing Alzheimer's.

And while measuring vitamin levels in blood is not at all a common practice, one group of researchers drew levels of vitamins B, C, D and E and found that patients with high blood levels of those vitamins had better global cognitive function than patients with lower levels of vitamins in their blood. But how do you know which foods you should be eating to get the proper levels of vitamins in your blood?

If you want the most bang for your nutritional buck, so to speak, the ORAC system can help clarify matters. A food's *ORAC*—or Oxygen Radical Absorbance Capacity—score measures the antioxidant capacities of various substances in the laboratory. Researchers have used the ORAC method, which was developed by the National Institutes of Health (NIH) and first published by the US Department of Agriculture (USDA) in 2004, to rank a huge range of foods, with certain spices, herbs, berries, legumes, and other plant-based foods taking top honors.

USDA researchers estimate that you can derive great benefits from consuming 3,000 to 5,000 ORAC units of antioxidants a day. In other words, it couldn't be easier to get your daily ORAC quota. Antioxidant-packed powerhouses are everywhere if only you know where to look.

To show you what I mean, let's start by examining those magic potions lurking in your spice cabinet. Did you know that the aromatic dried flower buds of an evergreen tree in the Myrtaceae family are among the chart-topping antioxidants of spices, with an ORAC score of 6,199 per ground teaspoon, or twice the minimum ORAC daily threshold? Native to Indonesia, this one little spice can do big things for your health. And, even better, chances are it's already sitting in your spice cabinet. Its common name? Cloves.

Here are the ORAC scores for a number of common herbs and spices, also measured in 100 grams.

HERB/SPICE	ORAC SCORE[5]
Cloves, ground	290,283
Oregano, dried	175,295
Rosemary, dried	165,280
Thyme, dried	157,380
Cinnamon, ground	131,420
Turmeric, ground	127,068

Other common herbs with beneficial ORAC scores include fresh marjoram (27,297) and dried parsley (73,670). We'll be using these power-packed herbs and spices as the basis for many of the recipes in the second part of the book.

So start spicing up your life, and your antioxidant intake will shoot through the roof. If you're not used to cooking with spices, trust me that your health—and your palate—will thank you for these little adjustments to your daily diet. Adding more beneficial spices to your favorite recipes will intensify the protective powers of your favorite foods—and their flavor, too.

Fruits and vegetables are important for so many parts of a properly functioning body, not least for infusing us with the antioxidants we need to fight off the reactive oxygen species that threaten to damage our cells. Preliminary findings from studies of animals and human blood suggest that a concentration of high-ORAC fruits and vegetables, like blueberries and spinach, in our diets can

HIGH-SPICE RECIPES

Herbed Pecans (page 118)

Strawberry Cinnamon Soup with Herbed Pecans (page 140)

Grilled Herbed Chicken Breasts with Sesame–Green Onion Rice and Bok Choy (page 176)

Curried Quinoa with Green Onions and Basil (page 199)

And all the recipes built around our delicious Brain-Boosting Broth (page 130) have a high spice content, including:

Curried Parsnip Soup (page 132)

Butternut Squash Soup with Miso (page 133)

Carrot-Ginger Soup (page 135)

Roasted Red Pepper Soup (page 136)

Sweet Corn and Poblano Chile Soup (page 137)

delay the aging process of our bodies and brains alike. And two human studies indicate that eating high-ORAC fruits and veggies can raise the antioxidant power of the blood between 13 and 25 percent.[6]

Here are just a few examples of brain-healthy foods from the main categories of antioxidants:

Vitamin C: Found in citrus fruits and their juices, berries, dark green vegetables (spinach, asparagus, green bell peppers, brussels sprouts, broccoli, watercress, other greens), red and yellow bell peppers, tomatoes and tomato juice, pineapples, cantaloupes, mangoes, papayas, and guavas.

Vitamin E: Found in vegetable oils (such as olive, soybean, corn, cottonseed, and safflower), nuts and nut butters, seeds, whole grains, wheat, wheat germ, brown rice, oatmeal, soybeans, sweet potatoes, legumes (beans, lentils, split peas), dark-green leafy vegetables, tomatoes, crabs, mangoes, and papayas.

Selenium: Found in Brazil nuts, brewer's yeast, oatmeal, brown rice, chicken, eggs, dairy products, garlic, molasses, onions, salmon, seafood, tuna, wheat germ, whole grains, and most vegetables.

Beta-carotene: Found in a variety of dark orange, red, yellow, and green vegetables and fruits such as broccoli, kale, spinach, sweet potatoes, carrots, red and yellow bell peppers, apricots, cantaloupes, and mangoes.

Polyphenols: Found in a wide variety of fruits (blackberries, blueberries, cantaloupe, cherries, cranberries, grapes, pears, plums, raspberries, and strawberries) and vegetables (broccoli, cabbage, celery, onion, and parsley), green tea, wine, and many other plants. The most abundant source of antioxidants found in plants, polyphenols can help protect tissues against free radicals and even have protective powers against problems as wide ranging as cardiovascular diseases, cancer, arthritis, and autoimmune disorders. They've been shown to inhibit plaque formation in the brains of transgenic mice (mice who have been genetically engineered to develop Alzheimer's changes in the brain), and might also restore *neuroplasticity*, which refers to the brain's ability to make new neural connections.

Flavonoids: Found in more than six thousand foods—virtually all plants—flavonoids are the polyphenol responsible for the brilliant red of strawberries, the deep blue of blueberries, and the cheerful orange of tangerines. If you're eating fruits and vegetables of any sort (the brighter, the better), you're likely to be getting your share of flavonoids, which function in the human body as antioxidants by helping to neutralize reactive oxygen species and to prevent them from damaging parts of cells. One of the best-known flavonoids is quercetin, which you can get in green tea, apples, grapes, and onions (especially red onions).

Is your head swimming yet? Not to worry. As the above lists indicate, antioxidants are pretty much everywhere you look; you can get them in a huge range of natural foods. But because of a phenomenon known as *bioavailability*—the capacity of the body to absorb the nutrients—it's best to consume antioxidants in the widest possible variety of foods because the bioavailability of nutrients from food sources varies widely by food type, and how the food is processed, prepared, and cooked. Since we don't yet fully understand why our bodies absorb some nutrients and expel others, scientists recommend that we play it safe by eating all sorts of different foods.

So, for their antioxidant content alone, you should build your diet around fruits and vegetables. Obviously, we're not saying that's *all* you should eat. Our approach is very inclusive, as our wide-ranging recipes indicate. You can continue to eat all of your favorite foods, but try to incorporate some good-for-you veggies

BETA-CAROTENE-RICH RECIPES

Butternut Squash Soup with Miso (page 133)

Super-Simple Ratatouille (page 185)

POLYPHENOL-RICH RECIPES

Blueberry-Banana Smoothie with Basil (page 95)

Soba Noodle Salad with Spicy Peanut Sauce (page 155)

FLAVONOID-RICH RECIPES

Beet Hummus with Feta and Basil (page 121)

Tomato and Arugula Salad with Parmigiano-Reggiano (page 145)

Beet and Melon Salad with Mixed Berries (page 153)

at every meal, with some flavorful spices sprinkled on top. If you're in the habit of having a hamburger three times a week, maybe cut that down to once and have a salmon burger on the other two days. It's all about making simple, straightforward substitutions. Again, even red meat, despite its high saturated-fat content, is fine in moderation, but remember that it's the side dishes—the spinach and the squash and the lentils—that are working hardest for your brain.

Regular consumption of fresh vegetables and olive oil—pillars of the antioxidant-rich Mediterranean diet, which I'll discuss in more detail in chapter 7—can significantly lower your oxidative stress and protect your brain against cognitive decline.[7]

Early evidence for the protective power of high-ORAC foods comes from rat studies. Rats fed daily doses of blueberry extract for six weeks before being subjected to pure oxygen suffered much less capillary damage in and around their lungs. In other tests, middle-aged rats were fed diets fortified with spinach or strawberry extract or vitamin E for nine months. A daily dose of spinach extract prevented some loss of long-term memory and learning ability normally experienced by fifteen-month-old

TOP ANTIOXIDANT FOODS (ORAC UNITS PER 100 GRAMS)

FRUITS		VEGETABLES	
Prunes	5770	Kale	1770
Raisins	2830	Spinach	1260
Blueberries	2400	Brussels sprouts	980
Blackberries	2036	Alfalfa sprouts	930
Strawberries	1540	Broccoli florets	890
Raspberries	1220	Beets	840
Plums	949	Red bell peppers	710
Oranges	750	Onions	450
Red grapes	739	Corn	400
Cherries	670	Eggplant	390

rats. Spinach also proved most potent in protecting different types of nerve cells in two separate parts of the brain against the effects of aging.[8]

As you can see, none of these are rare, hard-to-find foods; you can get them at every supermarket across the country. And if you occasionally want to take a break from our delicious vegetable recipes like Carrot-Ginger Soup (page 135) and Spicy Butternut Puree with Chinese Five-Spice and Honey (page 192), you can even get your antioxidant fix from legumes like small red beans, kidney beans, and pinto beans, all of which have sky-high ORAC scores.

Researchers in the Chicago Health and Aging Project found a link between vegetable consumption and a lower four-year risk of Alzheimer's.[9] Participants who consumed three servings of vegetables per day had a significantly lower risk of developing the disease than those who consumed less than one serving per day. All types of vegetable consumption were associated with a far slower rate of cognitive decline, but some are particularly beneficial, including sweet potatoes, zucchini and summer squash, eggplant, broccoli, lettuce, celery, apples, and—with the most dramatic impact of all—leafy greens like kale and collards. The Chicago Health and Aging Project researchers concluded that consuming two to four servings of leafy green, yellow, or cruciferous vegetables every day helped protect participants against age-related cognitive decline.

And in a thirty-year, longitudinal, population-based study recently published in the *Annals of Neurology*, researchers found that women who ate the most cruciferous and leafy greens showed a slower rate of cognitive decline than those who ate few or no veggies at all.[10] But interestingly, in this pool of more than thirteen thousand women, fruit consumption didn't seem to affect the rate of cognitive decline protection against the development of Alzheimer's disease. The reason for this discrepancy could be that vegetables generally have a higher concentration of antioxidants than fruit.

That said, blueberries and strawberries have consistently demonstrated protective antioxidant powers in the lab and in epidemiological studies, like the study of rats I mentioned earlier. Another recent study has shown that just *one cup* of berries can deliver all the antioxidants you need in a day. In general, orange, red, blue, and purple fruits, many of which are so-called superfruits—a category that includes dried cherries, acai fruit, and blueberries—tend to have the highest antioxidant content.

Drinking Your Way to Better Health

If you're not a fan of fresh fruits and vegetables, you can still get some of their nutritional benefits in liquid form. Fruit and vegetable juices, as well as wine, tea, and possibly even coffee, might all play an important role in delaying the onset of Alzheimer's disease, primarily because they all contain a powerful category of antioxidants known as polyphenols. *Polyphenols* are antioxidants exclusive to plants, and are the most abundant dietary antioxidants.

FRUIT JUICE

For all the claims made about acai and pomegranate juices over the last decade, even far more run-of-the-mill fruit and vegetable juices could protect nerve cells against hydrogen peroxide (a damaging reactive oxygen species). Recent clinical trials have demonstrated that drinking orange juice can reduce plasma concentrations of F2-isoprostanes, which is a biomarker of oxidative stress.[11]

And fruit and vegetable juices might be protective beyond their antioxidant content: many contain vitamins like folate, which has been associated with a decreased Alzheimer's risk. (See chapter 3, Vitamin B and the Brain, for more on the power of folate.)

While we don't yet know whether fresh fruit juices are superior to frozen or packaged juices, we can conclude that the presence of polyphenols have a protective effect. And recent in vitro studies (meaning cell-culture studies, or studies conducted in a Petri dish) demonstrate that many polyphenols protect mouse brain cells that have been isolated and grown in Petri dishes from oxidative stress.

In a population-based study of more than eighteen hundred Japanese Americans in King County, Washington, researchers tested whether consuming fruit and vegetable juices with a high concentration of polyphenols decreased Alzheimer's risk.[12] The study followed the participants, all of whom were dementia-free when the study

BRAIN-BOOSTING JUICES

Cantaloupe-Papaya Juice with Marjoram (page 92)

Cherry-Fennel Juice with Lime (page 92)

Spinach-Beet Juice with Citrus (page 93)

Sweet Peach Smoothie (page 96)

began, for up to nine years. After adjusting for potential complicating factors such as heart disease, the researchers found a 76 percent risk reduction for subjects who drank juices at least three times per week compared to those who consumed juice less than once per week. (The difference tended to be more pronounced among those with an APOE ε4 genotype and those participants who were not physically active.)

Some juices are better than others, of course, and there *is* a reason pomegranate juice has become such a favorite of health-food devotees over the last few years. Drinking it regularly has been linked to lowering the LDL cholesterol (low-density lipoprotein) and reversing arterial hardening, a known cause of heart disease and heart attacks. And a study from Loma Linda University suggested that administration of pomegranate juice to mice genetically engineered to develop Alzheimer's reduced the amount of toxic beta-amyloid protein (the plaque associated with Alzheimer's) found in the brains of these mice at autopsy.[13]

A HIERARCHY OF JUICES

Juices do contain nutrients, but they're also high in sugar; some are as sugary as soda. So it's best not to overdo it, and to stick to the juices with proven benefits.

The Good: These juices contain powerful antioxidants and can be a useful weapon in the fight against Alzheimer's.

- Pomegranate
- Acai
- Blueberry
- Concord grape

The Not-So-Good: While citrus juices contain high levels of the antioxidant vitamin C, they're neutral in terms of brain health, and too many added calories can add to the waistline.

- Orange
- Pineapple
- Lemonade
- Mango
- Cranberry (since most commercial brands come with added sugar)

GREEN TEA

Tea is the second most popular beverage in the world (after water), and it's also a major source of dietary flavonoids, a type of polyphenol that scientists have begun to study for potentially significant health benefits.[14] As a result of mounting epidemiologic evidence, they're focusing particularly on green tea—which has a high concentration of the flavonoid epigallocatechin-3-gallate (EGCG), an antioxidant that seems to be extremely effective at scavenging destructive free radicals—as a potential treatment for neurodegenerative disorders.[15]

And green tea exerts protective effects beyond its antioxidant properties: a recent study had more than one thousand elderly (seventy-plus years) Japanese participants complete a questionnaire that asked about the frequency of their green tea consumption.[16] The same participants underwent a commonly used memory test. When researchers compared the results of these tests with the participants' green-tea consumption, they found that the more green tea the participants consumed, the lower their rate of cognitive decline. The ones who drank two cups of green tea a day had dramatically lower rates of cognitive impairment than those who only drank three cups a week. Caffeinated and decaffeinated versions had similar health benefits.

While black tea and coffee didn't seem to exhibit the same protective benefits, neither beverage is without merit. Human epidemiologic and new animal data suggests that not only green but black tea, which is enriched in a class of flavonoids named *catechins*, might also help protect the aging brain.[17] (For more on coffee, see below.)

GREEN-TEA TREATS

Green Tea–Pomegranate Smoothie (page 93)

Green Tea Infused with Apples and Cinnamon (page 94)

Iced Green Tea with Pomegranate and Ginger (page 95)

RED WINE AND OTHER DRINKS MADE FROM GRAPES

Another beverage with unexpectedly powerful antioxidant properties is red wine, which has been shown to protect cardiovascular health and reduce the risk of developing Alzheimer's. But if you're not a fan of alcohol, don't fret: it isn't just Cabernet Sauvignon that can protect your heart and brain; Concord grape juice might be an equally powerful stand-in. Like wine, red and purple grape juice can help lower LDL cholesterol levels and blood pressure, and reduce your risk of blood clots.

The key protective ingredient in these grape-based drinks is *resveratrol*, a plant polyphenol that's found mainly in red wine and the grapes used to make them. Resveratrol might arrest the amyloid plaque development that occurs in Alzheimer's brains: a recent study in the *Journal of Biological Chemistry* suggests that resveratrol markedly lowers the levels of secreted amyloid peptide produced in different cells.[18] While resveratrol did not stop the production of amyloid, it did promote the degradation of the amyloid as well as activate the enzyme proteosome to break down other proteins. This activation process is promising, since amyloid plaque formation occurs years before Alzheimer's patients manifest symptoms. Long-term, preventive intake of resveratrol might help clear the amyloid peptide out of the brain before it ever forms a plaque, thereby delaying or even preventing the onset of Alzheimer's.

Red wine also contains *quercetin*, a flavonoid that's also found in garlic, onions, and apple skins. Quercetin has been shown to have anticancer properties and, in some studies, has been linked to a decreased risk in cognitive decline. In cell cultures, this compound reduces the amount of amyloid generated.

Not only that, but the increased levels of HDL (high-density lipoprotein) in the bloodstream that moderate alcohol ingestion produces, lowers cognitive risk by lowering confounding risk factors such as stroke and heart disease.

ALCOHOL AND BRAIN HEALTH

When it comes to alcohol, a little is good, but more is not better. Doctors recommend drinking no more than 30 grams of alcohol a day, which is the amount of alcohol in two 4-ounce glasses of wine, two beers, or two 1-ounce shots. Too much alcohol can poison both your liver and your brain, so do not exceed these guidelines. For brain health, the optimal dose is one to two glasses of red wine, or try our delicious Pomegranate Sangria (page 101) for something different. It's perfectly fine to drink this much on a daily basis provided you don't exceed this dose.

COFFEE

Coffee gets a bad rap sometimes, but a recent study found that it might be the number-one source of antioxidants in the American diet. And if that weren't enough, your daily cup of joe might also decrease your risk of getting Alzheimer's. In the Canadian Study of Health and Aging (CSHA), daily coffee drinking lowered Alzheimer's risk by 31 percent during a five-year follow-up; and the Finland, Italy, and the Netherlands Elderly (FINE) study likewise found drinking more than three cups a day of coffee was associated with the least ten-year cognitive decline among elderly men. The Three-City Cohort Study also indicated that this same quantity of caffeine (from both coffee and tea) was associated with a slower decline in verbal cognitive functioning among women but not men. Recent studies have shown that moderate coffee consumption—of dark-roast more than light-roast beans—is associated with a reduced risk of type 2 diabetes and Alzheimer's disease.[19]

Obviously, moderation is key here: chronic high doses of coffee can raise blood pressure and disrupt sleep. And the additives people put in coffee—particularly creamer, which often contains palm oil, and those sugary syrups—can also be a problem. But coffee taken black or with a little lowfat milk can be extremely good for you if you limit consumption to three cups a day. Or, to keep your caffeine content even lower, stick with decaf, which has the same antioxidant properties as regular coffee.

More recently, women with higher coffee consumption over a four-year period experienced less cognitive decline than those consuming little or no coffee. And the most convincing of the epidemiologic studies was one that showed that Alzheimer's patients consumed markedly less caffeine (based on dietary reporting) during the twenty years preceding diagnosis compared with age-matched individuals without Alzheimer's disease.[20]

CHAPTER 5

Inflammation: Turning Down the Heat in the Brain

I f you fall and injure yourself, the affected limb might swell in response—a sign that your body is releasing white blood cells and chemicals to repair body tissue. This is inflammation, and it can occur in almost any part of the body.

Inflammation is considered a normal physiological response to stress, our immune system's way of coping with injury or irritation. And while we can reduce the low levels of inflammation that accumulate over time by working out at the gym, higher levels of sustained inflammation can pose a grave threat to otherwise healthy tissues in the body.

Inflammation can also amplify already-existing damage, which can have potentially dangerous consequences. Inflammation is a feature of a variety of disorders including arthritis and other rheumatologic conditions, and neurological diseases such as multiple sclerosis. In some cases, the body loses its ability to regulate its own inflammatory reactions, which can damage tissues (joints in the case of rheumatoid arthritis, and nervous tissue in the case of multiple sclerosis).

More recently, inflammation has also been implicated in cardiovascular disease, obesity, and diabetes. Diet-induced obesity is associated with a chronic state of low-grade inflammation that can lead to insulin resistance, and that in turn can lead to type 2 diabetes.[1]

Even beyond the surprising links among diabetes, obesity, and Alzheimer's, inflammation plays a big role in the development of Alzheimer's disease, and post-mortem examination of Alzheimer's patients' brains has shown consistent inflammatory damage.[2] When inflammation occurs in response to deposits of beta-amyloid protein plaque (the protein associated with Alzheimer's) in the brain, the brain ages more rapidly. This can result in a condition known as chronic immune activation, which appears common in many cases of Alzheimer's.

Here's roughly how *chronic immune activation* works: When the brain produces amyloid plaque, cells in the brain called *microglia* recognize that the plaque shouldn't be there. The amyloid is a foreign substance that must be removed. In response, the microglia release inflammatory chemicals in an attempt to clear out the amyloid. Ultimately, though, the microglia are unable to remove the amyloid from the brain, and over time, both the amyloid and the inflammatory chemicals accumulate in the brain, a back-and-forth that leads to a chronic state of inflammation.

Think of it like a splinter wedged deep in your finger. Over time, the finger mounts an inflammatory response to remove or break down the splinter. If the splinter cannot be removed or broken down, the inflammatory response continues and the finger continues to swell.

Apart from the pathogenic, or disease-causing, role of immune responses, emerging evidence indicates that chronic inflammation is likely to compound, if not cause, the core pathological changes that occur in the Alzheimer's-affected brain. The key, then, is to reduce inflammation whenever possible. To do this, we must first understand the role that chronic inflammation plays in a number of different health conditions.

Diabetes and Dementia

It's an understatement to say that type 2 diabetes has been on the rise in recent decades. The World Health Organization estimates that 177 million people have diabetes worldwide, a figure that's likely to reach 300 million by the year 2025. According to the American Diabetes Association, in the United States alone, a new patient is diagnosed with diabetes every sixty seconds, adding to the 18 million patients nationwide and an estimated 9 million more that remain undiagnosed.

For our purposes, the inflammation that can lead to diabetes is important because epidemiologic studies have shown strong links between the risk of dementia and cognitive decline and an individual's history of diabetes. (I should note that these concerns only apply to type 2 diabetes, not type 1.)

Diabetes is a disabling condition that can severely damage the internal organs, particularly the kidneys, the eyes, and the nerves. It's a leading cause of heart disease, stroke, and kidney failure. If left untreated, it can also lead to lifelong debilitation in the form of dialysis placement, kidney failure, limb loss, and blindness.

But what exactly does diabetes have to do with Alzheimer's disease? The answer, scientists are discovering, seems to be a great deal. Links between abnormal insulin regulation or insulin resistance, both precursors of type 2 diabetes, and a person's risk of Alzheimer's disease have been borne out in numerous epidemiologic and clinical studies.

In cases of type 2 diabetes, the body makes plenty of insulin (the hormone responsible for getting sugar into cells) but the cells stop using insulin, so glucose (blood sugar) accumulates outside of cells instead of being transported into them. This leads to a state of chronic inflammation.

The brain needs a near-constant supply of glucose to keep it going, and insulin is a key player in providing it. Insulin is also responsible for regulating much of the activity within the brain cells themselves, as well as conveying signals from one neuron to the next. Because it's constantly transported across the blood–brain barrier, the levels of insulin found in the rest of the body tend to correlate with the levels found in the brain. It follows that when insulin and glucose metabolism are impaired, cognitive function likewise suffers.

One study has indicated that up to 43 percent of dementia cases could be attributed to diabetes, stroke, or a combination of the two.[3] Another study found that patients with borderline diabetes aged seventy-five or older had a 77 percent increased risk of developing Alzheimer's compared to patients who had normal blood-sugar levels.[4]

And not only that, but numerous studies have shown that *hyperinsulinemia*—a condition characterized by excess levels of insulin in the blood, and yet another consequence of insulin resistance and risk factor for type 2 diabetes—also carries a higher risk of Alzheimer's.[5]

The exponentially increasing prevalence of type 2 diabetes worldwide could mean that more and more people are also at risk for Alzheimer's. And a root cause of both these conditions is chronic inflammation. By eating the right foods and keeping our weight down, we'll be protecting our bodies from diabetes and our brains from degeneration.

Obesity and Alzheimer's

Even in cases where diabetes doesn't develop, new evidence indicates that obesity alone may play a significant role in cognitive decline and dementia, including Alzheimer's disease. This link has been demonstrated particularly when obesity first appears in middle age.

One of the seminal studies on obesity and Alzheimer's comes out of Finland, where researchers evaluated almost fifteen hundred people over a span of twenty years, measuring participants' body mass index (BMI) as well as cholesterol levels, blood pressure, height, and weight. The subjects were divided into three groups: those with a normal BMI (less than 25), those who were overweight (a BMI between 25 and 30), and those who had a BMI greater than 30.

The researchers found that obesity in midlife increased the risk for the developing dementia and Alzheimer's disease later in life. The participants who were obese in midlife were more than twice as likely to develop Alzheimer's disease later, even when smokers or those who suffered from high blood pressure or high cholesterol were not included in the group. When obesity was *added* to the profile of those who had both high cholesterol and high blood pressure, the risk of developing Alzheimer's increased up to sixfold, which suggests that, taken together, these risks could be used to predict whether or not the person would develop Alzheimer's.[6]

A study from the University of Washington confirmed the link between midlife obesity and dementia risk. Researchers evaluated five-year data on 2,798 participants from the Cardiovascular Health Cognition Study, a substudy of the Cardiovascular Health Study. The researchers measured the participants' weight and height at the time of their admission to calculate their present BMI.

To estimate their midlife BMI, participants were asked to self-report what they thought their weight had been at age fifty. With various complicating factors—age, race, sex, and education, as well as cardiovascular and dementia risk—all taken under consideration, researchers concluded that being obese at age fifty increased participants' risk of dementia by 40 percent.[7]

A study out of Sweden assessed the association between a higher BMI and an increased risk for dementia in twins and found that both being overweight and obese in midlife independently increased the risk of dementia and Alzheimer's disease.[8] In the Honolulu-Asia aging study, a higher BMI was associated with the risk of vascular (or stroke-related) dementia and other types of dementia in men, but not for Alzheimer's disease.[9]

These findings appear to hold true in the population at large. The Framingham study used MRI brain scans and found that people defined as obese as measured by a higher waist–hip ratio had a smaller hippocampus (the portion of the brain responsible for memory) and loss of total brain volume than people with lower waist–hip ratios.[10]

Researchers are still working to discover how exactly obesity can increase an individual's likelihood of developing Alzheimer's. A Kaiser Permanente study followed 10,276 people beginning from their mid-forties for over thirty years. The researchers looked at such factors as age, gender, race, education, smoking, alcohol use, diabetes, hypertension, and heart disease. They found that medically obese people—defined, you'll recall, as having a BMI over 30—had a 75 percent increased risk for developing dementia; whereas overweight people, with a BMI between 25 and 30, had only a 35 percent greater risk compared to people who maintained normal BMIs.[11]

Yet another Kaiser Permanente study performed a longitudinal analysis (an analysis of data gathered from a group of individuals studied over years, so that changes can be analyzed over time) of 6,583 participants who had their *sagittal abdominal diameter (SAD)*—or the amount of fat around their midsections—measured between the years 1964 and 1973. An average of thirty-six years later, researchers analyzed these same participants' medical records for dementia diagnoses. Overall, the study found that the participants with the top 20 percent SAD measurements in midlife were three times likelier to develop dementia than those in the lowest, a finding only mildly altered by adding BMI to the model. The investigators concluded that *central obesity*, or obesity in the abdominal region, in midlife increases risk of dementia independent of other conditions like diabetes or cardiovascular diseases.[12]

And that right there was the study's most intriguing finding: it wasn't just BMI, which measures the total fat level in the body, that mattered. It was *where* the fat was concentrated. Patients whose fat tended to settle at waist level (that is, those who were apple-shaped, or heavier in the middle) were 72 percent more likely to develop dementia later in life than those with greater concentrations of fat elsewhere (that is, pear-shaped people who are heavier in the bottom). Even participants whose BMI did not qualify them as overweight or obese, but whose fat was distributed disproportionately in the midsection, displayed a greater likelihood of developing Alzheimer's. Taken all together, these studies point to an incredibly nuanced relationship between body weight, fat distribution, and the onset of dementia. (If you're interested in knowing your sagittal abdominal diameter, your doctor can easily measure it. Just ask.)

Is Taking Anti-inflammatories the Solution?

Scientists first identified the connection between inflammation in the brain and Alzheimer's disease two decades ago, a discovery that proved a major landmark in our understanding of the biology of Alzheimer's. That finding led researchers to posit that nonsteroidal anti-inflammatory drugs, or NSAIDs, could be effective in treating Alzheimer's.

NSAIDs—which are found in a huge range of both over-the-counter and prescription medications such as ibuprofen (Advil and Motrin) and naproxen (Aleve)—are used to treat everything from toothaches to arthritis pain to fever. After uncovering the link between inflammation and Alzheimer's, researchers set out to prove that NSAIDs could also help in preventing or treating Alzheimer's, and indeed, tests on lab animals and large, population-based studies both showed promising results.

To name just a few: Researchers looked at data from the Rotterdam study and found a lower risk of Alzheimer's when test subjects took NSAIDs for at least two years.[13] The Cache County Study group reported similar findings in 2002: those who reported having taken NSAIDs for two years or more on a daily basis were less likely to develop Alzheimer's than those who didn't regularly take NSAIDs.[14] The longer participants used the NSAIDs, the lower their risk seemed to be.

Overall, a survey of more than twenty-five epidemiologic studies found that prior exposure to certain NSAIDs can decrease the risk of Alzheimer's, delay dementia onset, slow progression of the disease, and reduce the severity of cognitive symptoms. And in 2004, a genetic study showed that people taking NSAIDs were 36 percent less likely to develop Alzheimer's than family members not taking them. There's an important caveat, however: most of the studies surveyed found no benefit when NSAIDs were taken within two years of the onset of dementia, which suggests that timing is everything when it comes to NSAIDs exposure. Most epidemiologic data has repeatedly demonstrated that protracted use of NSAIDs *prior* to the onset of dementia can substantially lower the risk of developing dementia by 50 percent or more, especially in subjects carrying one or more genes associated with developing Alzheimer's.

This wave of epidemiologic evidence led researchers to investigate the efficacy of several different medications, including indomethacin (Indocin), diclofenac/misoprostol (Arthrotec), and rofecoxib (Vioxx), in treating Alzheimer's. Unfortunately, the results have been disappointing across the board. Clinical trials and other observational studies of various anti-inflammatories—including indomethacin, rofecoxib (the infamous Vioxx), naproxen (Aleve), and diclofenac (Voltaren)—have shown *no* results in treating Alzheimer's or mild cognitive impairment. Rofecoxib, which has since been withdrawn from the market, may have even accelerated cognitive decline in two of the trials.

It's possible that researchers need a much longer treatment period to show any positive results of the drugs or—what's even more likely—that the treatment is occurring too late, after the toxic amyloid has already accumulated in the brain, by which point reducing the inflammation would have no effect. And one study even found an association between heavy use of NSAIDs and *increased* amyloid accumulation.[15]

Another problem is that NSAIDs can seriously damage the kidneys and stomach if taken at high doses for long periods of time; they are, in fact, the most common cause of stomach ulcers. So if you're taking NSAIDs in an attempt to protect your brain from Alzheimer's, you might end up doing irreparable harm to your stomach or

APOE ε4: A GENETIC SUSCEPTIBILITY MARKER

The apolipoprotein E genotype is what's known as a genetic susceptibility marker. Carriers of certain types of the APOE gene, specifically ε4, are at a significantly higher risk of developing Alzheimer's. Having the APOE ε4 is hereditary, meaning either you did or didn't inherit it at the moment your parents conceived you. Though having the APOE ε4 allele (gene type) increases risk, we don't generally recommend that you get the genetic test (a blood test) unless you are having symptoms. This is primarily because of potential complications with insurance companies. Though the GINA act (Genetic Information Nondiscrimination Act of 2008) makes it illegal for insurance companies to discontinue insurance policies because of genetics, GINA excluded long-term care insurance. To ensure that patients get all the care they need, genetic testing should be limited to experts who can understand the information and counsel their patients accordingly.

kidneys in the process. There's even evidence that some anti-inflammatories, if taken continuously for a prolonged period of time, can elevate cardiovascular disease risk.

In light of these troubling findings, researchers have mostly abandoned studying NSAIDs for the treatment of Alzheimer's. And while we still hope that NSAIDs might be useful in preventing (if not treating) the disease, we don't yet have enough data to make meaningful recommendations.

So, if not through NSAIDs, how else can we reduce inflammation in our bodies, and without all the potential side effects? The answer is simple: through food. There's no better way to fight inflammation than by incorporating a few common, easily obtained ingredients into your daily diet.

What Do the South Asians Know That We Don't about Anti-inflammatories?

India has the lowest rates of Alzheimer's disease in the world. Studies done in South India, Mumbai, and the northern Indian state of Haryana have reported Alzheimer's rates ranging from about 1 percent in rural north India (the lowest anywhere in the world where Alzheimer's disease has been studied systematically) to 2.7 percent in urban Chennai.[16] Compare that to US rates of almost 10 percent.

This raises a major question: what do Indians know that we don't?

There are surely multiple reasons for this amazing statistic, including lower levels of underlying risk factors like the gene associated with Alzheimer's, and lower obesity rates than in the West (though diabetes rates are higher in India than here).

But there's another more isolated factor at play as well. After years of careful study, researchers have concluded that the Indian diet does play a crucial role in the country's remarkable avoidance of the Alzheimer's epidemic. It isn't just that Indians eat more fruit and vegetables and less saturated fat than we do, but that their diet regularly includes a disease-fighting agent called curcumin. And that right there might be the secret to South Asian's cognitive success.

Quite simply, curcumin (*Curcuma longa*) is a more-potent antioxidant than vitamin E, and a more-potent anti-inflammatory than ibuprofen. It works in part by turning off a protein that promotes an abnormal inflammatory response in the body. Curcumin also prevents platelets from clumping together to form blood clots, and is believed to lower cholesterol.

In a recent study conducted at the University of California at Los Angeles, scientists fed curcumin to laboratory animals bred to be prone to accumulate beta-amyloid plaque in their brains. The animals quickly performed better on memory tests than those on normal diets. But it was the internal examination that provided definitive proof, when researchers discovered that the curcumin blocked the accumulation of amyloid plaque and reduced the neural tissue inflammation related to Alzheimer's disease.[17]

If you're rushing over to the computer to see where you can buy this exotic and miraculous-sounding ingredient right this very moment, you can sit back down, because curcumin is neither rare nor exotic. In fact, you probably have some in your kitchen already.

Curcumin is the active ingredient in turmeric, the common spice that gives most curries their distinctive bright-yellow color. A powder ground from the root of a large-leafed Asian plant, turmeric has been the subject of no fewer than eight studies by the National Institutes of Health for its role in preventing not only Alzheimer's disease, but also cancer, cystic fibrosis, and arthritis. And none of these studies have identified any negative side effects of turmeric, either, so everyone can likely benefit from incorporating more turmeric into their daily diet. But how much more?

While the recommended therapeutic doses of turmeric vary, Dr. Andrew Weil suggests that adults can take between 1 to 3 grams of powdered dry root per day, 30 to 90 drops of fluid extract per day, or 15 to 30 drops of a tincture four times per day.[18]

Of course, the easiest and most complete way to obtain turmeric is in food. As always, daily intake—as opposed to sporadic meals that include large doses—is what matters in the long haul. And upping the amount of turmeric in your diet couldn't be easier.

TURMERIC RECIPES

Turmeric tincture, available in all health-food stores, is a fine additive to soups and broths, and it also tastes delicious in a plain cup of hot water and ginger. (In India, turmeric tincture is used as a gargle for sore throats, and is applied on bandages for wounds.) And turmeric tea is now on the shelves of every health-food store.

Eating spicy Indian curry once or twice a week could help prevent the onset of Alzheimer's disease and dementia. We've designed a number of recipes for spice lovers and more cautious palates alike. As you can see, we've provided you with a wide range of options.

Cinnamon

Another powerful Alzheimer's combatant that you'll find on your spice rack is cinnamon. Its mechanism for fighting Alzheimer's is slightly different from that of turmeric. As we discussed earlier in the chapter, diabetes is partially a result of increased insulin resistance, a condition that has been linked to Alzheimer's. Cinnamon works its magic by helping us regulate our metabolism and keep our insulin levels in check.

And while delicious cinnamon isn't, strictly speaking, an anti-inflammatory agent, numerous lab, animal, and human studies have shown that it can also alleviate factors associated with Alzheimer's disease by blocking and reversing tau formation in cell cultures that have been created to mimic the environment of the brain.

Let me explain. One major change that occurs in the brain of Alzheimer's patients is the accumulation of proteins called *neurofibrillary tangles*. These form within the brain's neurons rather than outside them, where the plaque develops. Neurons have arms called *axons*. Inside these axons are parallel proteins called *microtubules*. Just as railroad tracks are held together by railroad ties, microtubules are kept together with proteins called *tau*.

In Alzheimer's, the tau get all jumbled up, which leads to the microtubules becoming ensnarled. Researchers have learned that even before tau start clumping together with microtubules to form tangles, the structures inside the brain cells have already begun to change: when microtubule proteins become misshapen, they start to clump, causing all the molecules that move along the microtubules to back up because they cannot get past the clog. Cinnamon has been shown to reduce these blockages.

Cinnamon is being considered as a potential treatment for stroke for its ability to inhibit cell swelling. Laboratory studies also show that components of cinnamon control production of blood vessels that increase as cancer cells multiply and spread. Human studies involving control subjects and subjects with insulin resistance, hyperlipidemia (high blood cholesterol levels), hypertension (high blood pressure), and type 2 diabetes all show beneficial effects of cinnamon sticks and/or aqueous extracts of cinnamon on glucose, insulin, insulin sensitivity, lipids, antioxidant status, blood pressure, lean body mass, and gastric emptying. And cinnamon bark extract can inhibit viruses such as influenza, herpes, and HIV.

Perhaps most exciting of all, one new study reveals that cinnamon has direct anti-Alzheimer's properties, with an ability not only to inhibit the accumulation of the beta-amyloid plaque that leads to Alzheimer's disease, but to disassemble plaque that has already formed—meaning cinnamon might have both preventative and restorative properties.[19]

Not all studies have shown positive effects of cinnamon, though of course many different variables come into play, including the type and amount of cinnamon, and the other drugs subjects are taking. Still, it's pretty clear that something in cinnamon can help alleviate or even prevent the signs and symptoms of metabolic syndrome, type 2 diabetes, and cardiovascular and related diseases.[20]

Like most foods with anti-inflammatory properties, cinnamon is also a powerful antioxidant: a single teaspoon of this spice can fulfill our recommended daily allowance of antioxidants. And though you can get cinnamon extract in pill form, it's incredibly easy to work more of the spice into your diet. Sprinkle some on your morning oatmeal, or pinch a dab into your morning coffee or onto your afternoon snack of sliced apples.

Berries and Other Amazing Polyphenols

In the last chapter, we discussed the antioxidant qualities of polyphenols, but did you know that these miraculous compounds can be powerhouse anti-inflammatories as well? It's true. In a study of mice, polyphenols extracted from grapeseeds were shown to inhibit the buildup of amyloid plaque that can cause Alzheimer's, and to reduce inflammation in the brain.[21]

Another animal study looked at the role of the polyphenols in blueberries in reducing inflammation.[22] After exposing rats to the neurotoxin kainic acid, scientists gave blueberry extract to the animals. Another group of rats was fed a regular diet. The rats fed the blueberries recovered much more quickly from the neurotoxic exposure than the ones fed the control diet, which led scientists to conclude that polyphenols can have a powerful anti-inflammatory effect on the brain. They not only cushioned the brain damage caused by exposure to a neurotoxin, but they also might even have altered the expression of genes associated with inflammation. This means that external factors such as diet, illness, infection, trauma, inflammation, and a host of other events can more or less turn genes on or off, which is why inflammatory conditions are associated with the expression of certain genes.

Other research indicates that the polyphenolic compounds found in berry fruits, such as blueberries and strawberries, may protect our brains either by lowering oxidative stress and inflammation or by restoring how cells communicate with one another. They might also work by regulating the influx of ions such as calcium, which in turn prevents cells from becoming stressed and overly stimulated.[23]

And it isn't just berries. A wide variety of fruits and vegetables that contain antioxidants also have anti-inflammatory agents, and taken together, they're a powerful weapon in the fight against age-related neurodegenerative diseases such as Parkinson's disease and Alzheimer's disease. Increasing your dietary intake of fruits and vegetables can reduce your vulnerability not only to oxidative stress but to inflammation as well.[24]

BERRY RECIPES

Blueberry-Banana Smoothie with Basil (page 95)

Strawberry-Cinnamon Soup with Herbed Pecans (page 140)

Kale, Blueberry, and Pomegranate Salad (page 148)

Beet and Melon Salad with Mixed Berries (page 153)

As with so many aspects of Alzheimer's research, our understanding of both the antioxidant and anti-inflammatory qualities of dietary polyphenols remains incomplete. There's still a great deal we've yet to uncover about *bioavailability* (or how the body absorbs the nutrients), *biotransformation* (or the process by which a substance is altered inside the body), and many other factors. The most enduring mystery of all is how, or even if, the majority of these compounds cross the blood–brain barrier and reach the brain.[25] But as I said earlier, we can't sit around waiting for researchers to fill in the gaps in their knowledge. We need to start eating in a way that we know will benefit our brains and bodies—not next week or next year, but *today*.

CHAPTER 6

Fats:
The Bad, the Good,
and the Superior

For decades now, we've known that there are "good" fats and "bad" fats, but—as with so much else pertaining to our health—the data seems to shift daily, and sorting it all out can cause major headaches. But the classifications are really pretty straightforward when it comes down to it. Once we understand that dietary fats and oils from different sources have dramatically different impacts on our bodies, we can start making modest changes to our diets that will benefit our bodies and brains alike.

By cutting back on saturated fats (which often come from animal sources), eliminating trans fats (which are most commonly found in processed foods), and boosting our intake of polyunsaturated fatty acids (which derive from vegetable sources and fish), we can make substantial progress toward lowering our Alzheimer's risk.

Understanding Fat

Fat is, along with protein and carbohydrates, one of the three big categories of macro-nutrients that supply calories to the body. Fats, which are organic compounds made up of carbon, hydrogen, and oxygen, belong to a group of substances called lipids, and come in liquid or solid form. Though they can be an important energy source, the body prefers to break down carbohydrates for energy and store fats (unfortunately for us).

Though they've gotten a bad reputation in recent years, fats are absolutely essential for the proper functioning of the body. They maintain healthy skin and hair, as well as help the body absorb and move the vitamins A, D, E, and K through the bloodstream.

And last but not least, fats provide the essential fatty acids (EFAs) that the body can *only* obtain from food. Essential fatty acids are necessary for controlling inflammation, blood clotting, and brain development.

Are All Fats Created Equal?

Not at all. Some fats have beneficial properties and can reduce bad cholesterol (LDL) and raise good cholesterol (HDL). Other fats have harmful properties and can, among other things, promote atherogenesis (the development of blockages in arteries from the accumulation of lipids, cholesterol, and platelets). Atherogeneis is also associated with damage to the walls of blood vessels. In the heart, atherogenesis can cause blockages in the arteries, which ultimately result in heart attacks. A similar process in the brain leads to strokes.

Our diets contain mixtures of different fat types. Our goal is to alter our intake of fats in a way that promotes heart and brain health. According to the "Know Your Fats" page of American Heart Association website, we should

- "limit our total fat intake to less than 25 to 35 percent of . . . total calories per day;

- "limit saturated fat intake to less than 7 percent of total daily calories; and

- "limit *trans fat* intake to less than 1 percent of total daily calories.
- "The remaining fat should come from sources of monounsaturated and poly-unsaturated fats such as nuts, seeds, fish, and vegetable oils."[1]

Saturated fats and trans fats are the main categories of fats we need to avoid—and, unfortunately, they're found in the vast majority of commercially available foods these days: most animal products, partially hydrogenated oils, and many other processed foods.

Bad Fats

In addition to raising cholesterol levels, foods high in saturated fats might also contribute to cognitive decline. Therefore, cutting back on saturated fats and trans fats is one of the cornerstones of our Alzheimer's prevention program.

SATURATED FATS

In order to understand how fats differ, I should first explain that fatty acids are chains of carbon that can combine with other molecules. These acid chains vary in length and may be either saturated or unsaturated. Saturated fatty acids have adequate hydrogen molecules and therefore a straight configuration that allows them to pack into a solid crystal at ambient temperatures. The term *saturated fat* refers to a chemical composition with fatty acid chains that cannot incorporate additional hydrogen atoms. In other words, a saturated fat is one that's been fully saturated with hydrogen atoms.

Unsaturated fatty acids, by contrast, lack adequate hydrogen molecules, so rather than solidifying at ambient temperatures, they produce a liquid oil. Unsaturated fatty acids are labeled either monounsaturated or polyunsaturated depending upon the number of hydrogens which are missing. Polyunsaturated fatty acids (PUFAs) lack the greatest number of hydrogen, making them the most unstable.

Saturated fats are harder for the body to break down chemically than unsaturated fats, and so they tend to deposit more in the body, which leads to atherogenesis and myriad other health problems. Saturated fats have been long been implicated in high cholesterol, obesity, heart disease, stroke, cancer, and type 2 diabetes. And while the interactions among high-fat diets, cholesterol, obesity, genes, and Alzheimer's risk are fathomlessly complex, researchers now have reason to believe that dietary saturated fats might also affect memory function, and possibly increase people's risk of developing Alzheimer's disease.

Saturated fat is found mostly in foods from animals and some plants. Foods from animals include beef, beef fat, veal, lamb, pork, lard, poultry fat, butter, cream, milk, cheeses, and other dairy products made from whole and 2 percent milk, all of which contain dietary cholesterol. Foods from plants that contain saturated fat include coconut, coconut oil, palm oil and palm kernel oil (often called tropical oils), and cocoa butter.

Here are some of the biggest offenders in the saturated-fat category:

- High-fat dairy products (cheese, whole milk, whole-milk yogurt, cream, butter, and regular ice cream)

- Fatty fresh and processed meats (salami, sandwich meats, pastrami, mortadella, and other cured meats)

- The skin and fat of poultry

- Rendered animal fats (lard, shortening, tallow, suet)

- Butter

- Palm oil

- Coconut oil and dried coconut (though, as I'll discuss later, coconut fats also have unique benefits)

- Mayonnaise

The saturated-fat content of margarines and spreads is printed on the package or Nutrition Facts label. The same is true of chips, cookies, and most other packaged foods you buy at the grocery store. Increasingly, more restaurants and food purveyors, from Baskin-Robbins to Starbucks, are making this information more readily accessible both in brochures and online.

I'm by no means recommending that you shun these foods altogether. Ground liver, to name just one example, can also be a great source of brain-boosting B12, though whether the benefits of these vitamins offset the risks of the saturated fats remains dubious. If given the choice, opt for skim milk instead of heavy cream, skinless grilled chicken breasts over deep-fried chicken, and the salmon burger over the double bacon cheeseburger.

TRANS FATS

There is one category of fats, however, that have absolutely no place in our diets, and that's *trans-fatty acids (TFAs)*, also known as *trans fats*. Trans fats are monounsaturated or polyunsaturated fats that have been altered by partial hydrogenation. This process of partial hydrogenation forces the oils, which are naturally liquid at room temperature, to become solid, therefore modifying the fat so that it resembles a saturated fat. While trans-fatty acids are considered unsaturated by chemical definition, the transformation is so severe that trans fat cannot be legally labeled as monounsaturated or polyunsaturated fat on packages.

Trans fats also resemble saturated fats in that they can raise "bad" and lower "good" cholesterol levels, and like saturated fats they've been linked to heart disease. Trans fats have zero health benefits and contain no essential fatty acids. While some animal fats (from cows and sheep, for example) naturally contain small amounts of trans fats, most of the trans fats that we consume today are artificially engineered. They're found in hydrogenated or partially hydrogenated vegetable oils that form when vegetable oil hardens, a process called *hydrogenation*. Foods containing hydrogenated oils have a

HOW TO AVOID TRANS FATS

Start cooking primarily with olive oil, and check nutritional labels to make sure there are no trans fats in the processed foods you buy at the supermarket. And while you're at it, try to minimize the number of processed foods you're taking home in the first place. Instead of chips, grab a bag of trail mix (especially trail mix with berries) or some string cheese. Instead of cookies, try some almonds, dried cranberries, or a bag of lowfat granola. You can now buy bags of delicious goji berries at most health-food stores, and even mainstream grocery stores now stock pomegranate seeds in convenient, grab-and-go containers. These are all great snacking options.

longer shelf life than their natural counterparts, and often don't require refrigeration. The most common foods that contain trans fat include these:

- Hard margarines and shortenings
- Commercially fried foods (fried chicken)
- Some commercial baked goods (donuts, cookies, and crackers) and cake mixes
- Soup cups
- Frozen foods (pies, pot pies, fish sticks, frozen pizzas)

TFAs are also formed during the process of hydrogenation, making margarine, shortening, cooking oils, and the foods made from them a major source of TFAs in the American diet. Partially hydrogenated vegetable oils provide about three-fourths of the TFAs in the US diet. In clinical studies, TFAs or hydrogenated fats tended to raise total blood cholesterol levels. Some scientists believe they raise cholesterol levels more than saturated fats. TFAs also tend to raise LDL (bad) cholesterol and lower HDL (good) cholesterol when used instead of natural oils. These changes may increase the risk of heart disease.

Keep trans-fat intake to less than 1 percent of total calories. For example, if you need 2,000 calories a day, you should consume less than 2 grams of trans fat, or about half a teaspoon. As with saturated fats, you can check your trans-fat intake by studying the Nutrition Facts label of your favorite foods at the grocery store and increasingly at restaurants as well.

The Fat-Alzheimer's Connection

We've already discussed the links among obesity, diabetes, and Alzheimer's; let's look more closely at some of the mechanisms at work here. A number of studies have shown that a high intake of saturated fatty acids and high-cholesterol foods can increase risk of cardiovascular disease and therefore of cognitive decline and Alzheimer's disease. A high-fat diet can also lead to insulin resistance and oxidative stress, both of which, as we've seen, can accelerate the development of Alzheimer's disease.

Most, but not all, evidence of this link comes from animal studies in which mice and rats were fed diets of different fat levels and then given learning and memory tests. In one such study, scientists fed one group of mice genetically engineered to develop Alzheimer's a diet high in saturated fat and cholesterol, and another control group of mice a diet without these fats. After two months, when both sets of mice were tested for memory-related tasks, the ones that had been fed the saturated fats couldn't remember, much less perform, the tasks, and the control group could. When their brains were examined, the scientists found increased levels of the toxic beta-amyloid protein in the mice fed the high-saturated-fat diet.

Rats and mice are obviously not humans, and we can't draw definitive conclusions about human pathology from such studies—and, as I've pointed out elsewhere, we cannot conduct similar tests on humans for a host of biomedical and bioethical reasons. We also don't know if it's the saturated-fat intake alone or the corollary health conditions that arise from the high-fat diets that are causing the rats' memory problems. Still, despite these caveats, we *can* induce from these rodent tests that diets high in saturated fat have an effect on cognitive ability.

Complicating this conclusion, however, are the findings of the Rotterdam population study that found no association between high levels of saturated-fat intake and an increased risk of dementia. But in yet another study, researchers found that people who were APOE ε4 carriers (one of the apolipoproteins, or blood proteins that carry fat and cholesterol in the blood and to and from the liver, associated with Alzheimer's) and who had also high intakes of saturated fat had an increased risk of developing of Alzheimer's disease, especially when compared with APOE ε4 carriers who had a lower intake of saturated fat.[2] Unsaturated fats, on the other hand, didn't appear to influence the odds of developing Alzheimer's disease among either ε4 carriers or noncarriers.

As these contradictory findings indicate, the jury is still out on the exact relationship between saturated fats and Alzheimer's. Even if Alzheimer's weren't such an incredibly complicated disease, it's always a challenge to isolate cause and effect in studies of human diets. Still, the incomplete evidence we do have makes a convincing case to replace animal-based saturated fats with healthier vegetable- and marine-based unsaturated fats.

But it bears repeating that you don't have to ban saturated fats from your diet altogether. There's absolutely nothing wrong with splurging on a cheeseburger every once in a while; red meat is a great source of essential B vitamins. The key is to strike the right balance, and the best way of doing this is to practice moderation. It's fine to eat high-fat meats and fully loaded ice-cream sundaes every once in a while, just not every day (or even every week).

And there are even some saturated fats that you should go out of your way to eat regularly. While coconut and avocados both contain high saturated fat, they can also be beneficial to your health. That's because they're what's known as a *medium-chain fatty acid (MCFA)*. We metabolize each fatty acid according to its size, so even though coconut oil's and avocados' physiological effects are distinctly different from those long-chain fatty acids found in meat, milk, and eggs, we should limit our intake to one serving per day because avocados and coconuts are both high in saturated fats.

Medium-chain fatty acids may also provide an added energy source for brain cells (in the form of an energy source called a ketone)—a discovery that may prove important in treating Alzheimer's since we know that Alzheimer's-afflicted brain cells don't get sufficient nourishment.

Good and Superior Fats: The Fats Your Body Needs

It's important to remember that not all fats are bad. Some are essential for keeping your brain and body functioning properly, and these are the ones we need to incorporate into our diet.

UNSATURATED FATS

An *unsaturated fat* is a fat or fatty acid with at least one double bond within the fatty acid chain. Where double bonds are formed, hydrogen atoms are eliminated. Thus, a saturated fat has no double bonds and the maximum number of hydrogens bonded to the carbons. Unsaturated fat molecules contain somewhat less energy (that is, fewer calories) than an equivalent amount of saturated fat. They're liquid at room temperature and come from plants such as olive, peanut, corn, cottonseed, sunflower, safflower, and soybean.

Unsaturated fats contain those essential fatty acids our bodies need to thrive but, unlike saturated fats, they don't raise blood cholesterol; they actually tend to lower the level of cholesterol in the blood. (Trans fats are the big exception here: as mentioned earlier, they might be unsaturated, but they're also completely without health benefits.)

Unsaturated fats are found in natural (that is, not hydrogenated) vegetable oils, especially olive and canola oils; nuts and seeds; avocados; and many fish (the fattier the better). Most animal fats contain both unsaturated fats and saturated fats in varying proportions.

There are two big categories of unsaturated fats, *monounsaturated fats* and *polyunsaturated fats*. This refers to the number of double bonds in the fatty acid chain: monounsaturated fats have one double bond, while polyunsaturated fats have multiple double bonds. Both of these types of fats may help lower your blood cholesterol level and possibly improve your cognitive function when you use them in place of saturated and trans fats. For optimum brain health, strive to replace most saturated fats and *all* trans fats with polyunsaturated fatty acids and monounsaturated fatty acids. Let's look at the unsaturated fats in more detail.

Monounsaturated fatty acids (MUFAs). Studies suggest that the higher the proportion of monounsaturated fats in our diet, the lower our risk for coronary heart disease. Monounsaturated fats are found in nuts and high-fat fruits such as olives and avocados. The best source of MUFAs is olive oil, which is about 75 percent monounsaturated fat. And a recent study called the Three-City Cohort Study found that participants who used olive oil with regularity (both in cooking and in salad dressing) showed lower risk of cognitive decline for visual memory compared to participants who didn't use olive oil.[3] Other natural oils—grapeseed, peanut, sesame, corn, safflower, canola, and sunflower, among others—are also good sources of MUFAs. These oils also contain polyunsaturated fats.

Polyunsaturated fatty acids (PUFAs). And now, at last, we come to the "magnificent" fats. Far and away the brain-healthiest fats you can consume are polyunsaturated fats, or *polyunsaturated fatty acids*, which are found in leafy greens, seeds, and nuts. Vegetable oils such as soybean oil, corn oil, canola oil, and cottonseed oil, and many kinds of nuts are good sources of polyunsaturated fats.

But the most important source of PUFAs is fatty fish, which contain omega-3s, the most critical fatty acid for brain health. In fact, by eating just one meal of fish per week, you reduce your risk of Alzheimer's disease by somewhere between 40 to 60 percent. That's right: a single meal is all it takes.

What Are Omega-3s?

Omega-3s are a category of polyunsaturated fatty acids that are crucial to the development and maintenance of many central-nervous-system functions. Along with the PUFAs, omega-3s, omega-6s, and omega-9s are the building blocks for hormones that control immune function, blood clotting, and cell growth as well as components of cell membranes. (The numbers refer to where the carbon chain has its first double valence bond: in omega-3s, it's three carbons from the beginning; in omega-6s, it's between the sixth and seventh carbon atoms; in omega-9s, it's between the ninth and tenth. These differences on a molecular level all affect the body differently.)

There are two critical omega-3s that the body needs for maintenance, structure, and function of many organs and tissues: *eicosapentaenoic acid (EPA)* and *docosahexaenoic acid (DHA)*.

DHA (docosahexaenoic acid) in particular is essential to the integrity of brain cells, the demise of which is a hallmark of Alzheimer's disease. While the findings have been more mixed in humans, studies done on aged animals have shown DHA to play an important role in preserving memory and possibly also slowing the development of Alzheimer's. (And slowing Alzheimer's is a fine goal: if the age of onset is delayed to 100, few of us will live to develop it; delay it until age 120, and no one will.)

Eating more foods containing omega-3s is a cornerstone of any Alzheimer's-prevention protocol for the simple reason that we can only obtain these essential fatty acids from our diet; our body doesn't produce them on its own.

How to Get Omega-3s in Your Diet

Modern diets have very few sources of omega-3 fatty acids, which are primarily found in the fat of coldwater fish such as salmon, tuna, sardines, herring, mackerel, black cod, and bluefish. Eggs and poultry also contain omega-3s, though in lesser quantities.

Some plant-based foods—such as walnuts, flaxseeds, spinach, canola and other vegetable oils, and wheat germ—contain the omega-3 precursor *alpha-linolenic acid (ALA)*, which the body must convert to EPA and DHA. Many of these vegetarian sources, however, especially the vegetable oils, are also high in omega-6 fatty acids, the consumption of which we must be careful to moderate.

The Omega-3–Omega-6 Balance

The body constructs hormones from both omega-3 and omega-6 fatty acids. In general, hormones derived from the two classes of essential fatty acids have opposite effects. Those from omega-6 fatty acids tend to increase inflammation (an important component of the immune response), blood clotting, and cell proliferation, while those from omega-3 fatty acids decrease those functions. To maintain optimum health, both families of hormones must be in balance.

These days especially, that's easier said than done. While omega-3s can require some effort to work into our diets, omega-6s—which are present in most seeds and nuts, and the oils extracted from them—are abundant, perhaps overabundant. In fact, refined vegetable oils (like soybean oil) that contain omega-6s are used in so many processed and fast foods that as much as 20 percent of all calories in the American diet might come from this source. (Olive oil, by contrast, is a MUFA and therefore doesn't contain omega-6s—yet another reason to make it an everyday staple.)

Many nutrition experts believe that before we relied so heavily on processed foods, humans consumed omega-3 and omega-6 fatty acids in roughly equal amounts. These days, though, many of us get as much as fourteen to twenty-five times more omega-6s than omega-3 fatty acids. This imbalance between omega-3s and omega-6s has been linked to the rise of a wide range of diseases, including asthma, coronary heart disease, many forms of cancer, autoimmune and neurodegenerative diseases, and may also contribute to obesity, depression, dyslexia, and hyperactivity.

Omega-3s and Alzheimer's

Restoring the balance between omega-3s and omega-6s in our bodies—which almost always means increasing our intake of the former—can go a long way toward improving our overall health. But can a higher intake of omega-3s really protect our brains? Epidemiologic studies point to a possible association between dietary intake of omega-3 fatty acids and reduced risk of cognitive decline and dementia.

The Chicago Health and Aging Project (CHAP) used dietary surveys to assess omega-3 fatty acid levels in participants' diets. Researchers computed weekly fish consumption and administered simple and complex memory tests over an average of four years. After adjusting for a multitude of factors, investigators found that participants who ate fish at least once a week had a rate of cognitive decline 10 percent slower than those who ate less than one fish meal per week, and 12 percent slower among those who ate at least two or more fish meals per week. Still, because they were simultaneously studying other protective dietary habits, the CHAP researchers couldn't conclusively isolate fish consumption as the reason for this decline.[4] The apparent dementia-delaying properties of fatty fish could be a result of a generally healthy diet in addition to the omega-3 fatty acids in fish. And even if it *is* the fish, other potentially protective ingredients could also play a role: for example, in addition to omega-3s, fish is also a good source of the antioxidant selenium, and

THE BEST FISH FOR BRAIN HEALTH

- Anchovy
- Bluefin
- Halibut
- Herring
- Mackerel
- Salmon
- Sardine
- Trout, rainbow
- Tuna

fatty fish is also rich in vitamin D, which is essential for neurological function and also has antioxidant and anti-inflammatory properties.

While, granted, we need to perform a great deal more research on this subject, we have seen repeatedly that regular fish-eaters experienced reduced cognitive decline and a slower loss of memory function than those who ate less fish. Other large population-based studies have supported the hypothesis that fish consumption can significantly boost neurological function. In the Cardiovascular Risk Factors Aging and Dementia (CAIDE) Finland study, higher saturated-fatty-acid intake in midlife was associated with lower cognitive function, more impaired memory, and an increased risk of mild cognitive impairment, while higher intake of polyunsaturated fatty acids was associated with better semantic memory (or understanding of concepts), and frequent fish consumption was associated with both better semantic memory and overall cognitive function. And across the board, populations with elevated fish consumption experience a lowered risk of cognitive decline.[5] Still more evidence: patients already diagnosed with Alzheimer's have lower levels of DHA as well as lower levels of the omega-3 fatty acids.[6] And recent data from the OPAL study suggested that higher fish consumption is associated with better cognitive function in later life.[7]

So even if we don't yet fully understand the precise mechanisms by which fish protects our brains, we can definitively conclude that a high intake of omega-3 fatty acids is essential for both neural cognitive development and normal brain functioning. We have very little to lose—and everything to gain—by eating more fatty fish.

What Protects: A general rule of thumb when it comes to fish and the brain: The fattier, the better. In the Cardiovascular Health Cognition Study, fatty fish such as tuna was associated with a lower risk of developing dementia whereas lean fried fish was not.

FISH RECIPES

Ahi Tuna on Rye with Spinach Pesto Yogurt (page 158)

Sautéed Trout with Wilted Watercress and Oyster Mushroom Salad (page 163)

Striped Bass with Golden Tomato and Sweet Pepper Stew (page 165)

Arctic Char with Grilled Red Onion (page 166)

Grilled Salmon with Molasses-Lime Glaze (page 167)

Salmon and Vegetables Steamed on Banana Leaves (page 168)

Grilled Salmon with Cherry Tomato Salad and Green Beans (page 170)

Caponata (page 212)

- Tuna salad (as long as it contains little mayonnaise, since most brands are loaded with saturated fat)

- Sushi made with tuna, salmon, herring, mackerel, halibut, or trout

- Halibut steaks

- Grilled salmon and salmon burgers

- Lox and other smoked salmon

What Doesn't Protect: White fish such as cod—the fish used in most frozen and fast-food fish entrees—has a low DHA content, and when it comes to protecting the brain, fish that's high in DHA seems to have the most risk-reduction properties.

- Most boxed fish sticks from the supermarket, which are usually cod-based and therefore low in DHA

- Fish and chips

- Most fried-fish takeout/fast food

VEGETARIAN SOURCES OF OMEGA-3S

- Flaxseeds (also known as linseeds)
- Soybeans
- Spinach
- Tofu
- Walnuts
- Wheat germ

CHAPTER 7

The Mediterranean Diet: Full-Package Protection against Alzheimer's

The Mediterranean diet deliciously encapsulates all the beneficial ingredients and eating trends we've been discussing. This diet—which gets its name from the dietary habits of people in countries bordering the Mediterranean Sea, specifically Greece, Italy, Turkey, and Spain—is built around the fruits and vegetables that grow in abundance in this part of the world. It's also rich in whole grains, potatoes, beans, nuts, seeds, and, perhaps most central of all, MUFA-rich olive oil. Mediterranean people also drink red wine on a daily basis, but always in moderation (defined as two 4-ounce glasses a day) and primarily at mealtimes.

Given these countries' proximity to the sea, fish—the ultimate lean protein, and the best possible source of those all-important omega-3 fatty acids that work so hard for our hearts and brains—is another key ingredient in Mediterranean diet. Other than fish, though, the animal-based elements are scant: Mediterranean-diet adherents usually consume fewer than four eggs a week, have a low to moderate consumption of both red meat and poultry, and eat only a little dairy, usually in the form of yogurt.

In short, the red meat and dairy products that are the source of most saturated fats in the typical American diet just don't get top billing in Mediterranean countries. One of the principal differences between the Mediterranean diet and the typical modern American diet is this lower level of saturated fats and the higher levels of "good" fats such as those monounsaturated and polyunsaturated fatty acids found in fish, nuts, and olive oil. Still, though, researchers increasingly believe that the efficacy of the Mediterranean diet resides not in any single ingredient, but in how the various foods and nutrients combine in our bodies.

Mediterranean Meals and the Brain

Now that we know more or less what the Mediterranean diet is, let's examine more closely why so many health experts recommend we adopt it. Numerous studies have shown that this plant- and fish-based diet can protect against a number of major health conditions and diseases, including obesity, cardiovascular disease, hypertension, high cholesterol, and cancer. And research has proven that people who regularly consume olive oil—the essential ingredient of the Mediterranean diet—have a lower risk of not only heart disease but also osteoporosis and rheumatoid arthritis. But though olive oil can lower cholesterol levels and protect against heart disease, it's still calorically dense, and Mediterranean diners never overdo it. Moderation in all things is always the keynote of this type of eating.

While researchers have historically focused mostly on the Mediterranean diet's impact on heart health, recent studies have shown that eating this way can protect our brains as well. People who adhere to the Mediterranean diet have lower rates of obesity and diabetes, both of which, as we've seen, can be linked to cognitive decline. Another example: antioxidants protect us from Alzheimer's, and red wine, the Mediterranean beverage of choice, contains high levels of the antioxidant resveratrol. Leafy green vegetables like kale and spinach that are popular in Mediterranean countries contain high levels of B vitamins, which are crucial for maintaining brain health.

It doesn't stop there: Mediterranean people eat a great deal of fish, and the polyunsaturated fatty acids in fish have been shown to protect cognitive health as have the monounsaturated fatty acids in olive oil. The concentration of fruits, vegetables, olive oil, and wine in the Mediterranean diet also help reduce inflammatory markers, including white-blood-cell counts, associated with Alzheimer's. And while the whole grains and complex carbohydrates like chickpeas and cannellini beans that people in Mediterranean countries consume have no direct anti-Alzheimer's properties, they do help keep insulin levels more in check than the white bread and refined grains Americans tend to prefer, which means they help protect against diabetes and, by extension, Alzheimer's.

Even the way people in Mediterranean people prepare foods contributes to their overall health. Fish and chicken tend to be grilled; our fondness for deep-frying everything is unheard-of on the shores of the Mediterranean. Other popular Mediterranean food-preparation methods include baking and sautéing, both of which maximize the flavor while minimizing the fat.

In short, almost every ingredient that researchers have isolated as brain-beneficial also happens to be a traditionally "Mediterranean" food. There really is a remarkable degree of overlap, and quite a few targeted studies bear out the link between Mediterranean-style eating and slower cognitive decline, a reduced risk of developing mild cognitive impairment (MCI), reduced risk of progression from MCI

LIFESTYLE COMPONENTS OF THE MEDITERRANEAN DIET

An enjoyment of food—which we have too often lost in this country, and which the delicious recipes in part 2 aim to promote—is another important element of the Mediterranean diet. People sit down for their meals, and eat them with their families. They do not consume food while driving to work or standing on the corner. Mediterranean people also tend to linger over their meals for hours, a lifestyle habit that promotes a healthier relationship with food and tends to keep the weight off. It may seem counterintuitive, but the more we pay attention to and enjoy what we're eating, the less likely we are to overconsume.

Another cultural aspect of Mediterranean-style eating is that family life tends to revolve around the kitchen, unlike the TV room where far too many Americans spend their time. In Mediterranean countries, there's a tradition of children learning to cook with their parents, passing down recipes from one generation to the next, so they understand the importance of delicious and healthful food from an early age.

to Alzheimer's, and a decreased risk for Alzheimer's and reduced all-cause mortality among patients who already have Alzheimer's.

Researchers in New York City closely tracked more than twenty-two hundred dementia-free individuals for up to thirteen years, gathering medical and neurological histories, performing physical and neurological examinations, and conducting detailed dietary surveys and memory tests with each participant. After scoring each participant's diet based on the Mediterranean elements it contained (and taking all sorts of other risk factors and/or protective behaviors like physical exercise into consideration), researchers found that the higher a participant's Mediterranean diet score, the lower his risk of developing Alzheimer's and the slower his rate of cognitive decline in general.[1]

Perhaps the most interesting aspect of this study was the credence it gave to the whole-diet theory—that is to say, the acknowledgment that the combination of these foods often conferred more health benefits than any single ingredient in isolation. The researchers concluded that consuming all or at least many elements of this diet confers more health benefits than consuming any single nutrient in isolation, or attempting to cover the same bases in a multivitamin.

The Three-City Cohort Study also demonstrated that adherence to the Mediterranean diet led to slower rates of cognitive decline, though these researchers didn't focus explicitly on Alzheimer's disease or incident dementia, meaning the dementia that developed over the course of the study. Another report from this study found that participants consuming diets high in fruits, vegetables, fish, and omega-3 fatty acids had decreased incidence of all-cause dementia and Alzheimer's compared with those whose diets were lower in these foods and nutrients.[2]

A recent report from the Washington Heights–Inwood Columbia Aging Project (WHICAP) found a lower risk of Alzheimer's associated with diets characterized by higher intakes of oil- and vinegar-based salad dressing, nuts, fish, tomatoes, poultry, cruciferous vegetables, fruits, and dark and green leafy vegetables in conjunction with a lower intake of high-fat dairy products, meat, and butter—in other words, all the major elements of the Mediterranean diet.[3]

The Cache County Study on Memory and Aging found that participants who ate more fruits, vegetables, whole grains, nuts, fish, and low-fat dairy products had higher cognitive function than when they enrolled in the study and experienced less cognitive decline over eleven years of follow-up than those who ate these foods less regularly.

But though there've been many studies, only one clinical trial has explicitly analyzed dietary patterns in relation to cognition or Alzheimer's risk. The Dietary Approaches to Stop Hypertension (DASH) diet is rich in fruits, vegetables, and low-fat dairy foods and low in saturated fat, total fat, and cholesterol. In a recent randomized clinical trial of 124 participants with elevated blood pressure who were sedentary and overweight or obese, subjects on the DASH diet exhibited more neurocognitive improvements than others.[4]

Understanding how the Mediterranean diet—or any composite diet, for that matter—affects us is an extremely nuanced undertaking. The dominant reasons cited for the Mediterranean diet's protective qualities are moderate consumption of alcohol; low consumption of meat and meat products; and high consumption of vegetables, fruits, nuts, omega-3 fish oils, olive oil, and high-fiber legumes, but very few studies have looked at the big picture of how all these ingredients interact synergistically in our bodies.

MEDITERRANEAN SIDE-DISH RECIPES

Sautéed Mushrooms with Spinach and Black Vinegar (page 187)

Spaghetti Squash with Carmelized Onion and Cilantro (page 191)

Spicy Butternut Squash Puree with Chinese Five-Spice and Honey (page 192)

Roasted Carrots (page 194)

MEDITERRANEAN MAIN-DISH RECIPES

Ahi Tuna on Rye with Spinach Pesto Yogurt (page 159)

Sautéed Trout with Wilted Watercress and Oyster Mushroom Salad (page 163)

Super-Simple Ratatouille (page 185)

Wild Rice with Root Vegetables (page 200)

Red Lentils with Kale and Miso (page 202)

Compared with the traditional single-food or nutrient recommendations we've focused on throughout this book, the whole-diet or dietary pattern approach is more complicated, especially since it's also possible that moderate lifestyles in general, which obviously vary according to different cultural environments, protect from cognitive impairment. People who exercise regularly, who drink in moderation and eat more vegetables than meats, have better overall health outcomes than others: healthier physiques, healthier hearts, and yes, healthier brains. But it's important to remember that—since we haven't yet definitively identified all the nutrients that drive these benefits—it's adhering to this diet *in its totality* that appears to be protective. So it's important to adhere to all its elements rather than picking and choosing a few at random. That's why the recipes in part 2 combine multiple brain-healthy ingredients rather than focusing on one or two in isolation. We are trying to teach you a new way of cooking and thinking about food that will protect your body and brain for many decades to come.

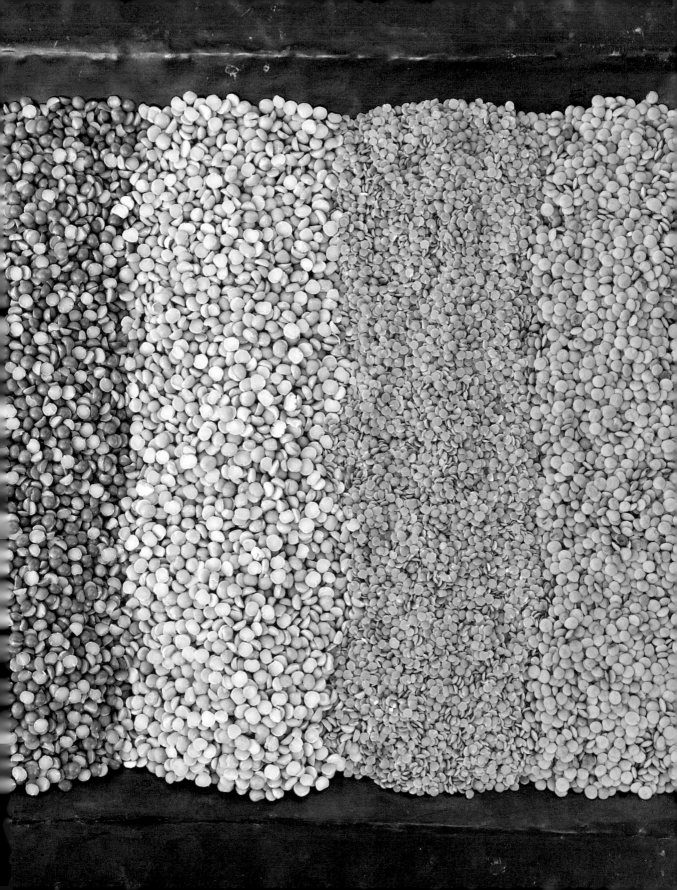

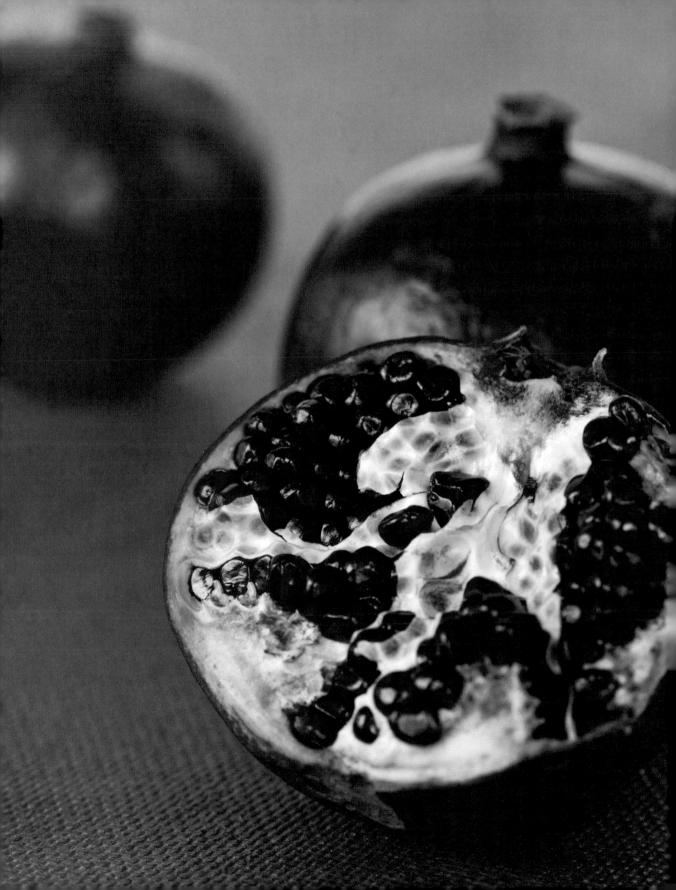

RECIPES FOR
BRAIN
HEALTH

Change your eating habits, and you'll change your health. And yes, it will take an initial investment of both time and money, but once you stock up on what you'll need, you'll be ready to cook. After you buy some easy-to-find herbs, spices, and kitchen appliances, you'll make a minimal monthly investment in groceries. We'll provide a shopping list, including turmeric, good organic tea, quinoa, and an inexpensive coffee grinder that will be used to grind spices. All can be obtained at your local supermarket, food co-op, Indian spice store, well-stocked health-food store, or online. We'll also tell you what types of foods don't belong in your kitchen.

Here's your shopping list.

Equipment

Inexpensive coffee grinder for grinding spices. Whenever possible, we recommend that you buy whole spices and grind your own. Buying whole spices, which are available in most health-food stores, is preferable for several reasons. First, grinding them fresh ensures a stronger flavor and increases the potency of the spice, which in turn increases its health benefits as well. You can also be assured that whole spices don't have any mysterious additives like some store-bought packaged spices. Last but not least, whole spices stay fresher longer, and like fresh-ground coffee, they taste better, too. After just a few days of grinding your own spices, you'll wonder why you ever settled for the preground variety.

Juicer. A juicer really is a great piece of equipment to have in your home kitchen. It allows you to make fresh fruit and vegetable juices, which are extremely healthy. You can then blend these juices with other ingredients to create killer shakes and smoothies. You can get a great juicer for under one hundred dollars—Hamilton Beach makes a relatively inexpensive one that works on harder vegetables such as carrots and cucumbers as well as soft, ripe fruits.

Blender. Many makes and models are available for less than seventy-five dollars. Any home blender that can be used to make a margarita will work for the recipes in this book. For the drink and smoothie recipes, you can substitute a blender for a juicer if necessary, but be advised that a puree made in a blender will be thicker than juice made with a juicer. You can add a bit of water to the mixture to adjust the consistency.

Food processor. A food processor is particularly helpful for making dressings, dips, and side dishes. The capacity needed for a food processor depends on what you need to do with it. Larger processors are better for making smoothies and dough, whereas smaller processors are good for chopping and grinding herbs. Typically, a nine-cup processor is very versatile. It is also good to get a high-powered food processor because the motor is less likely to burn out.

Pantry Staples

- Whole grains, including brown rice and quinoa
- Legumes, including lentils, split peas, chickpeas, and all types of beans
- Honey (without preservatives or chemical additives of any sort)
- Nuts, including walnuts, pecans, hazelnuts, and pistachios
- Seeds, including pumpkin and sunflower

Spices and Herbs

- Turmeric (ground)
- Liquid turmeric
- Curry powder
- Garam masala powder
- Cinnamon (ground)
- Cinnamon sticks

- Cloves
- Parsley (fresh and dried)
- Rosemary (dried)
- Thyme (dried)
- Marjoram (dried)

Produce

- Fresh garlic
- Onions
- Leafy green vegetables including spinach, kale, and bok choy
- Asparagus
- Romaine lettuce and other salad greens
- Mushrooms (particularly shiitake and crimini)

- Tomatoes
- Eggplant
- Dried tart cherries
- Dried acai berries
- Dried cherries
- Fresh blueberries (when in season)
- Fresh strawberries (when in season)
- Pomegranates (when in season)

Fish

- Tuna (canned)
- Salmon
- Halibut

Beverages

- Turmeric tea
- Organic green tea
- Organic black tea
- Pomegranate juice
- Red wine

Pantry Detox

Here's what to ditch:

- Lard and butter
- All high-fructose corn syrup sweeteners
- Anything containing high-fructose corn syrup sweeteners, including sports drinks
- Soda made with anything more than sparkling water and fruit juice
- White bread
- White rice
- Oversized juice glasses
- Anything containing hydrogenated or partially hydrogenated oils

Here's what to put on the back of the shelves and learn to use sparingly. Like high-fructose corn syrup, these foods can promote obesity and insulin resistance, which ultimately contributes to the risk of developing diabetes, a known risk factor for Alzheimer's.

- White flour
- Sugar
- Cornstarch

And now let's get cooking!

Introduction from Chef Beau

I've always valued cookbooks for their aesthetic qualities—the beautiful photographs and recipes provide inspiration and ideas for putting food on the table—but I never thought of them as important tools. And I certainly never really imagined that I'd have the opportunity to help people improve their lives through a book. Then one day at Sanctuary, I met Dr. Marwan Sabbagh, and he asked me if I would be interested in working with him on this book. It's such an awesome concept: improve your brain health by changing the way you eat. And the smart dietary choices you make not only influence your brain health, they have an impact on your entire body as well. By choosing nutritious, quality ingredients, you can prepare meals that taste great and that make you—and those around you—healthier from head to toe. I knew I had to be a part of this project. It was a no-brainer, pardon the pun.

A FEW COOKING TIPS

- Get to know your purveyors. In the produce department, grocers are often willing to help you determine the ripeness and readiness of fruit and vegetables. In the meat section, they can advise you on the appropriate cuts and portion sizes.

- Salt and pepper are a must for great recipes. The phrase "salt to taste" should be taken as an overall approach when cooking any recipe. Many dishes will call for salt and pepper to be added, while others may not. The choice to add salt and pepper is subjective and depends solely on your palate. Salt and pepper measurements do not need to be exact, and you should rely on your own personal taste preferences to determine how much to add. Start with a little, have fun while you cook, and taste as you go.

- Choose organic whenever possible. It's healthier for your brain and you as a whole.

Drinks

Cantaloupe-Papaya Juice with Marjoram

In this super-healthy, refreshing drink, ripe fruit is absolutely essential. Choose a cantaloupe that's very aromatic and not too firm. The papaya should also have a little give: when gently pressed into the fruit, your finger should leave an imprint. Smell the papaya near the stem end of the fruit; it should be richly fragrant. Cantaloupe is a good source of polyphenols, and nutmeg contains good amounts of vitamins A and C and choline. The spice also has small amounts of thiamin, riboflavin, niacin, vitamin B6, and folic acid. Marjoram, with its high ORAC score (see page 39), is an excellent source of antioxidants, and is a great finish to this beverage. **MAKES 1½ CUPS**

1 ripe papaya (about 1 pound), peeled, seeded, and chopped

½ ripe cantaloupe, peeled, seeded, and chopped

½ cup ice cubes

Pinch of ground nutmeg

Sprig of marjoram, for garnish

Combine the papaya, cantaloupe, ice, and nutmeg in a blender and puree until smooth.

Pour into a glass and garnish with the marjoram. Serve right away.

Cherry-Fennel Juice with Lime

Sweet and tart cherries, a good source of polyphenols, give this drink a great color and real character. Fennel, a common ingredient in the Mediterranean diet, has antioxidant properties because it contains quercetin, but Beau likes it simply for its wonderful licorice-like qualities. Fresh lime juice provides a nice shot of vitamin C. **MAKES 3 CUPS**

2 cups cherries, stemmed and pitted

½ cup ice cubes

1 cup chopped fennel bulb, plus fennel fronds for garnish

2 tablespoons freshly squeezed lime juice

Combine the cherries and ice in a blender or food processor and puree until smooth. Strain the puree through a fine-mesh sieve into a pitcher, pressing on the solids to extract as much juice as possible.

Push the chopped fennel through a juicer. Add the fennel juice to the cherry juice, and then whisk in the lime juice. Pour into glasses and garnish with fennel fronds. Serve right away.

Spinach-Beet Juice with Citrus

This brain-healthy drink contains two vegetables that are high in polyphenol anti-oxidants. Citrus juices contain a rich source of vitamins, minerals, and dietary fiber, which are essential for normal growth and development and overall nutritional well-being. It has been discovered that citrus may also help to reduce the risk of many chronic diseases. A few of the health benefits of coriander include treatment of swellings, high cholesterol levels, anemia, digestion, and menstrual disorders. You can grate in a little bit of fresh ginger for an added kick. **MAKES ABOUT 1 CUP**

2 cups baby spinach, plus
  1 leaf for garnish
1 medium beet, chopped
1 tablespoon freshly squeezed
  orange juice
1 tablespoon freshly squeezed
  grapefruit juice
1 teaspoon freshly squeezed
  lemon juice
1/2 teaspoon coriander seeds,
  toasted and ground in a
  spice mill

Chill the serving glass in the freezer.

Push the spinach through a juicer, followed by the beet. Combine the juices in a pitcher and stir in the coriander seeds with the orange, grapefruit, and lemon juices.

Pour into the chilled glass and garnish with the spinach leaf. Serve right away.

Green Tea–Pomegranate Smoothie

Green tea has a soothing, almost floral scent that contrasts nicely with the acidity of the pomegranate. This smoothie, with its wonderful ying and yang elements, is absolutely delicious. Matcha refers to finely milled or fine-powder green tea with a high concentration of antioxidants. When drunk regularly, it can boost metabolism and even help reduce cholesterol levels. Compared to regular yogurt, Greek-style yogurt is lower in sodium and carbohydrates and is high in protein, which helps promote fullness. Pomegranate juice packs tons of antioxidants. **MAKES ABOUT 2 1/2 CUPS**

1 cup plain Greek-style yogurt
1 ripe banana, peeled and
  chopped
1/4 cup honey
1/4 cup pomegranate juice
2 teaspoons matcha
  (green-tea powder)
1 cup ice cubes

Combine all of the ingredients in a blender and puree until smooth.

Pour into glasses and serve right away.

Green Tea Infused with Apples and Cinnamon

This drink is as brain healthy as beverages get. It starts with green tea, a great source of EGCG catechins (see page 46), which are among the most potent antioxidants. Cinnamon, with its very high ORAC score, is also rich in antioxidants. When shopping, look for locally grown apples that are in season. **MAKES ABOUT 3 CUPS**

3 cups water

1 green tea bag

½ stalk (bottom portion) fresh lemongrass

3 apples, peeled, cored, and chopped

1 cinnamon stick

Fresh mint sprigs, for garnish

Bring the water to a gentle boil in a small saucepan. Turn off the heat and add the tea bag. Bruise the lemongrass with the back of the blade of a chef's knife and add it to the pan. Let steep for 30 minutes, and then pour the tea through a fine-mesh sieve into a clean saucepan. Add the apples and cinnamon and bring to a boil over high heat. Turn down the heat and simmer until the apples are fork tender, about 6 minutes.

Using a slotted spoon, remove and discard the cinnamon stick and apples. Pour the tea into cups or mugs, garnish with the mint, and serve right away.

Iced Green Tea with Pomegranate and Ginger

The trick to this delicious drink is to make the tea with water that has been infused with fresh ginger. You can use less ginger for a milder taste, or leave the ginger in during the tea-steeping time for a spicier flavor. Pomegranate is an excellent source of antioxidants, while ginger is known to be very effective in alleviating symptoms of gastrointestinal distress. For extra-powerful gingeriness, grate the ginger instead of slicing it. **MAKES ABOUT 1 QUART**

1 quart water

2-inch piece fresh ginger, peeled and sliced

5 green tea bags

3 tablespoons honey

1 cup pomegranate seeds

2 tablespoons blueberry-pomegranate juice

Ice cubes, for serving

Bring the water to a boil in a small saucepan. Add the ginger to the water, remove the pan from the heat, and let steep for 10 minutes.

Add the tea bags to a heatproof pitcher. Pour the ginger-infused water through a fine-mesh sieve into the pitcher. Add the honey and pomegranate seeds and let steep for 5 minutes.

Remove and discard the tea bags. Stir in the blueberry-pomegranate juice and serve over ice.

Blueberry-Banana Smoothie with Basil

This recipe supports brain health because it includes blueberries, which are high in polyphenols, and fresh basil, a good source of flavonoids. Both basil and yogurt are staple ingredients in the Mediterranean diet. The molasses gives the smoothie a subtle sweetness and caramel taste. You can vary this recipe by using pineapple juice or pomegranate juice in place of the orange juice. **MAKES 2¹/₂ CUPS**

1 pint fresh blueberries

2 ripe bananas, peeled and chopped

1/4 cup plain Greek-style yogurt

1/4 cup freshly squeezed orange juice

2 tablespoons molasses

1/2 cup ice cubes

1/4 cup chopped fresh basil leaves, plus sprigs for garnish

Combine the blueberries, bananas, yogurt, orange juice, molasses, and ice in a blender and puree until smooth.

Transfer the mixture into a bowl or pitcher and stir in the basil. Pour into glasses, garnish with basil sprigs, and serve right away.

Sweet Peach Smoothie

The key to this recipe is using a ripe, in-season peach. Here in Arizona, we get amazing peaches from the farms in the city of Queen Creek, as well as from Utah. It's always good to get to know the produce guys at your local grocery store because they will tell you when peaches are in their prime. Peaches contain numerous nutrients that are good for your body, including niacin, thiamin, potassium, and calcium. They are also high in beta-carotene, which promotes healthy hearts and eyes. The darker the peach's color, the more vitamin A it has in its pulp. Peaches may also help in maintaining healthy urinary and digestive functions. There's some evidence that flaxseed oil, which is a good source of omega-3 fatty acids, may help reduce your risk of heart disease, cancer, stroke, and even diabetes. **MAKES ABOUT 3 CUPS**

1½ cups apple juice

1 ripe peach, peeled, pitted, and chopped (about ³/₄ cup)

³/₄ ripe banana, peeled and chopped

1 tablespoon vanilla yogurt

6 ice cubes

2 teaspoons honey

2 teaspoons flaxseed oil

Combine the apple juice, peach, banana, yogurt, and ice in a blender and puree until smooth. Add the honey and flaxseed oil and puree briefly to incorporate.

Pour into glasses and serve right away.

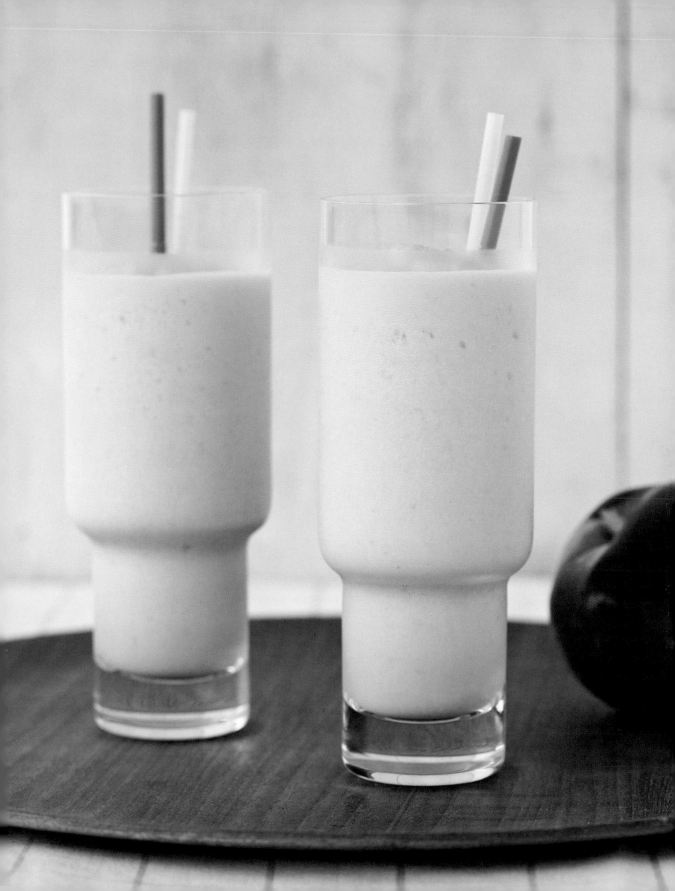

Banana-Kale Wake-Up Smoothie

If you don't have a juicer, you can simply throw the kale leaves into the blender along with the other ingredients and puree. Or you can finely chop the kale by hand and stir it in after blending. Either way, you'll have a thick smoothie with a slightly crunchy texture that drinks like a meal. Kale is high in polyphenols; its subtle bitterness is nicely balanced by the sweetness of the bananas. Ground cloves have a very high ORAC score and are a great source of antioxidants (see page 39). But go easy on the clove garnish—its flavor and aroma are potent. MAKES 2 CUPS

½ cup chopped kale leaves

2 ripe bananas, peeled and chopped

½ cup plain Greek-style yogurt

¼ cup freshly squeezed orange juice

1 tablespoon honey

½ cup ice cubes

Ground cloves, for garnish

Push the kale through a juicer. You should have about 2 tablespoons of kale juice.

Combine the kale juice, bananas, yogurt, orange juice, honey, and ice in a blender and puree until smooth.

Pour into glasses, garnish with a tiny pinch of ground cloves, and serve right away.

Avocado and Asian Pear Smoothie with Ginger

Asian pear, which is high in vitamin C, and ginger, a good source of vitamin B6, are a classic combination, and the avocado adds a little richness that binds together the ingredients in this recipe. Though this smoothie tastes deliciously rich and creamy, it's actually low in saturated fat and cholesterol. Added brain-health benefits are the riboflavin (vitamin B2) and vitamin C in the coconut water and the antioxidant properties of the rosemary. MAKES 2 CUPS

1 Asian pear, peeled, cored, and chopped

1 ripe avocado, pitted, peeled, and chopped

¾ cup coconut water

5 ice cubes

2 teaspoons peeled, grated fresh ginger

⅛ teaspoon chopped fresh rosemary

Combine all of the ingredients in a blender and puree until smooth.

Pour into glasses and serve right away.

Tropical Ginseng Smoothie

The tropical flavor of this smoothie comes from the fruits as well as the macadamia nuts. If you can't find fresh ripe mangoes, use pineapple juice in place of the mango juice and chopped pineapple instead of the chopped mango. For many centuries, the Chinese have used ginseng for energy. It can also help with stress and assist in fighting off infections. This recipe is a delicious and healthy way to take in vitamin E.
MAKES ABOUT 2½ CUPS

2 mangoes, peeled and chopped

½ ripe banana, peeled and chopped

¼ cup unsalted macadamia nuts, toasted and chopped

½ teaspoon ginseng powder, preferably Korean white ginseng

2 tablespoons plain yogurt

1 ice cube

6 fresh mint leaves, plus sprigs for garnish

3 fresh strawberries, hulled, plus more for garnish

Push half of the mango pieces through a juicer. You should have about 1 cup of juice.

Combine the mango juice, remaining half of the mango pieces, banana, macadamia nuts, ginseng powder, yogurt, and ice in a blender and puree until smooth.

Add the mint leaves and strawberries and puree just until incorporated.

Pour into glasses. With a paring knife, slit the strawberries for garnish and slip one onto the edge of each glass. Garnish with mint sprigs and serve right away.

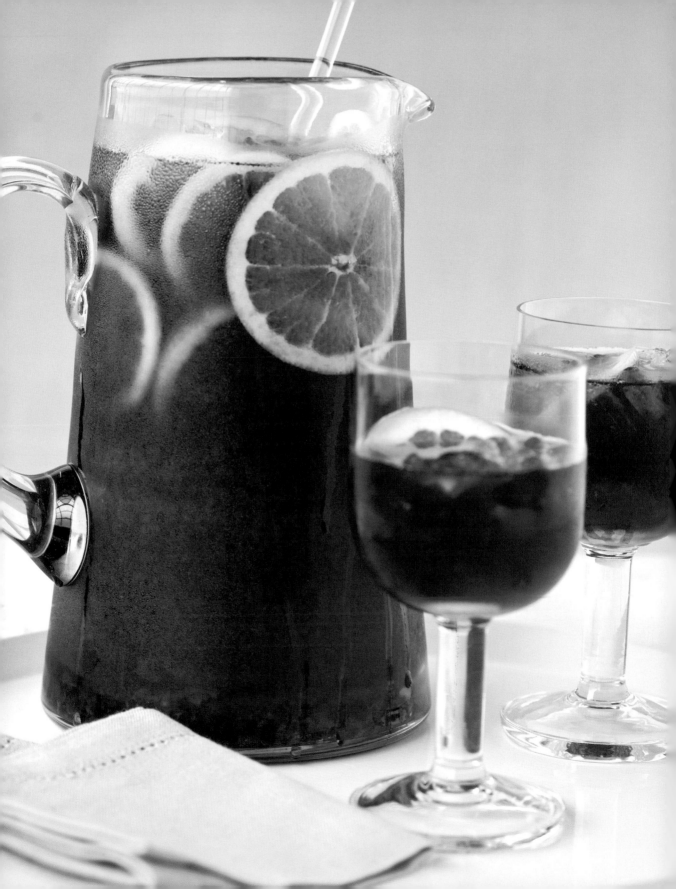

Pomegranate Sangria

If Dr. Sabbagh thinks red wine is good for the brain, Chef Beau isn't going to argue. This is a super easy recipe. All it takes is some mixing and pouring. Pomegranates contain resveratrol, just like red wine does (see page 47). **MAKES ABOUT 2½ QUARTS**

1 (750 ml) bottle Cabernet Sauvignon (or other red wine)

2 cups sparkling water

1 cup pomegranate juice

1 cup freshly squeezed orange juice

½ cup honey

¼ cup freshly squeezed lemon juice

2 tablespoons Grand Marnier (or other orange-flavored liqueur)

1 cup pomegranate seeds

1 lemon, sliced into thin rounds

1 orange, sliced into thin rounds

4 cups ice cubes

Combine the wine, sparkling water, pomegranate juice, orange juice, honey, lemon juice, Grand Marnier, pomegranate seeds, lemon slices, and orange slices in a large pitcher and stir to blend in the honey. Add the ice and serve.

Five-Spiced Three-Pear Smoothie

Chef Beau likes to use Bartlett pears, Asian pears, and Seckle pears in this recipe. You can use other varieties, but make sure that they are tender and fully ripe. Pears are a great antioxidant and are great for people who suffer from food allergies. They are also excellent for the prevention of heart disease. The smoothie strikes a perfect flavor balance of sweetness and spice, and texture is silky smooth thanks to the frozen yogurt. Serve it any time of the day, even as a great finish to a healthy dinner. **MAKES ABOUT 1½ CUPS**

1 ripe Bartlett pear, peeled, cored, and chopped

1 ripe Asian pear, peeled, cored, and chopped

1 ripe Seckle pear, peeled, cored, and chopped

1 cup vanilla yogurt

2 tablespoons freshly squeezed lemon juice

1 teaspoon Chinese five-spice powder

2 thin slices Asian pear, for garnish

Fresh mint sprigs, for garnish

Combine the chopped pears, frozen yogurt, lemon juice, and five-spice powder in a blender and puree until smooth.

Pour into glasses, garnish with pear slices and mint sprigs, and serve right away.

Breakfasts

Not-Your-Average Steel-Cut Oatmeal

Chef Beau's grandfather, who lived into his late nineties, started every morning with a bowl of steel-cut oatmeal. He recommended that his grandson do the same: "You have to eat your porridge, boy," was his advice. This recipe is not your grandfather's oatmeal—it's a tricked-out version, one that's both tastier and more brain-healthy than plain old porridge, though it is a time-intensive recipe. The raisins are packed with polyphenol antioxidants and the pistachios provide a dose of vitamin E. With all the flavor and texture in this oatmeal, you won't be tempted to load it down with butter or cream, which means less saturated fat. **MAKES 4 SERVINGS**

6 cups nonfat milk

Seeds from 1 vanilla bean, split lengthwise

1 teaspoon ground coriander

1/4 cup maple syrup

1 1/2 cups steel-cut oats

2 tablespoons shelled raw pistachios, toasted and chopped

1/2 cup golden raisins

1/2 cup unsweetened shredded coconut, toasted

Pour the milk into a medium saucepan over medium-high heat, and bring to a boil. Add the vanilla seeds, coriander, and maple syrup. Stir in the oats and bring back to a boil, and then turn down the heat to maintain a simmer. Cook, uncovered, stirring occasionally, until the oats are tender, about 1 to 1 1/2 hours.

Spoon the oatmeal into individual bowls; garnish with pistachios, raisins, and coconut; and serve right away.

Elemental Granola

This recipe is a house favorite at Elements, Chef Beau's restaurant. Granola is as fun to make as it is to eat. It's also quite versatile. You can enjoy it with cold milk as cereal, layer it with fruit and yogurt to make parfaits (see pages 106 and 108), or simply eat it out of hand as a snack. Whole grains, like the oats in this recipe, are high in fiber and are important elements in the Mediterranean diet. This granola is also chock full of nuts and seeds that provide vitamin B6 and vitamin E, nutrients that support brain health. In addition, the dried cherries, cranberries, or blueberries that add color and tangy flavor are rich in polyphenol antioxidants. Chef Beau likes to use "razz cherries" in his granola; they're dried cherries that have been infused with raspberry juice. Razz cherries are large and plump, so if you decide to try them, chop them before mixing into the granola. MAKES ABOUT 7 CUPS

6 tablespoons maple syrup
6 tablespoons brown sugar
1/4 cup vegetable oil
1 tablespoon vanilla extract
1 teaspoon ground cinnamon
1/2 teaspoon salt
3 cups old-fashioned oats
1/2 cup sesame seeds
1/2 cup raw whole
   macadamia nuts
1/2 cup shelled raw pistachios
1/2 cup sliced almonds
1/2 cup dried tart cherries,
   cranberries, or blueberries
1/2 cup sweetened shredded
   coconut

Preheat the oven to 250°F. Line a baking sheet with parchment paper.

In a large bowl, stir together the maple syrup, brown sugar, oil, vanilla, cinnamon, and salt until well combined. Add the oats, sesame seeds, macadamia nuts, pistachios, and almonds and stir until the ingredients are evenly coated. Spread the mixture into an even layer on the prepared baking sheet and bake until evenly golden on top, about 1 1/4 hours, stirring every 20 minutes or so.

Let the granola cool on the baking sheet. Add the dried cherries and coconut and toss to combine. The granola will keep in an airtight container at room temperature for up to 1 month.

Banana, Granola, and Yogurt Parfaits

Chef Beau prefers these parfaits made with Elemental Granola (page 105) because it adds an especially crunchy texture and great coconut flavor. Be sure to use Greek-style yogurt in this recipe—its consistency is much richer and thicker than regular yogurt—and opt for a low-fat or nonfat version to keep the saturated fat to a minimum. The sunflower seeds add supplemental crunch and nutty flavor as well as vitamins B6 and E. This recipe can easily be doubled. MAKES 2 SERVINGS

1 cup low-fat or nonfat plain
   Greek-style yogurt
2 tablespoons shelled raw
   sunflower seeds, toasted
1 tablespoon honey, plus more
   for drizzling
2 ripe bananas, peeled and
   sliced thin
1/2 cup granola

In a small bowl, stir together the yogurt, 1 tablespoon of the sunflower seeds, and the honey.

Spoon 1/4 cup of yogurt into the bottom of two serving dishes or parfait glasses. Sprinkle 2 tablespoons of granola into each dish and top with one-quarter of the banana slices. Repeat the layering using the remaining yogurt, granola, and bananas. Drizzle the parfaits with honey, sprinkle with the remaining 1 tablespoon of sunflower seeds, and serve right away.

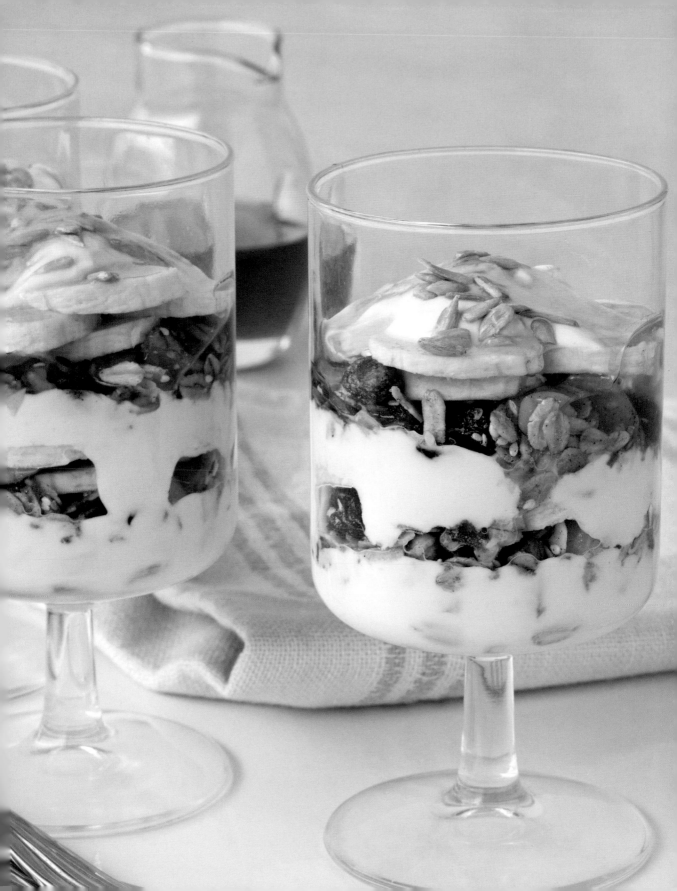

Stone Fruit Parfaits with Minted Yogurt

The plum, cherries, grapes, and prunes not only add color and flavor to these parfaits, they're also rich in brain-healthy polyphenol antioxidants. The orange is included for flavor and color contrast and for added vitamin C. If you like, sprinkle some Elemental Granola (page 105) or the granola of your choice over the parfaits just before serving to give them some textural interest and grainy, nutty goodness.

MAKES 2 SERVINGS

1 small orange

1 ripe, firm plum, pitted and coarsely chopped

1 cup sweet red cherries, pitted and coarsely chopped

1 cup seedless red grapes, halved

1/4 cup pitted prunes, coarsely chopped

1/2 cup freshly squeezed orange juice

2 tablespoons freshly squeezed lemon juice

2 cups low-fat or nonfat plain Greek-style yogurt

1/2 cup chopped fresh mint leaves, plus 2 sprigs mint for garnish

1 tablespoon honey

Cut off the top and bottom of the orange and set the fruit on a cut end. Working from top to bottom and following the contour of the orange, use a sharp knife to trim away the peel with the pith in strips, rotating the fruit after each cut. Hold the fruit in your hand and make a pole-to-pole cut between the membrane and the flesh of each section to free the orange segments. Add the segments to a medium nonreactive bowl, along with the plum, cherries, grapes, prunes, orange juice, and lemon juice. Toss to combine, cover, and refrigerate for 2 hours to allow the flavors to blend.

In a small bowl, mix together the yogurt and chopped mint and let stand at room temperature for 1 hour.

When ready to serve, pour off the liquid from the fruit mixture. Spoon 1/2 cup of the yogurt into the bottom of two serving dishes or parfait glasses, and then top each with one-quarter of the fruit mixture. Repeat the layering using the remaining yogurt and fruit. Drizzle each parfait with honey and garnish with a mint sprig.

Corn and Crab Omelet with Avocado

This simple omelet is great for breakfast or brunch, but it also makes a terrific light lunch or dinner, and it's elegant enough to serve to company. The vegetables and avocado are good sources of numerous vitamins, and the red bell pepper and onion supply polyphenol antioxidants that support brain health. If you want to inject some spiciness into the dish, add some minced jalapeño chile to the aromatic vegetables while they sauté. MAKES 1 OMELET, SERVING 2

2 ounces Dungeness or lump crabmeat (1/4 cup)

4 large eggs, beaten

Salt and freshly ground black pepper

4 tablespoons extra-virgin olive oil

1/4 cup fresh corn kernels or frozen thawed corn kernels

1 tablespoon finely diced red bell pepper

1 tablespoon finely diced red onion

1 green onion, white and green parts, chopped

1/2 ripe avocado, pitted, peeled, and sliced, slices fanned

1 lemon wedge

Pick through the crabmeat, removing any shell and cartilage fragments.

Heat a medium nonstick skillet over medium-high heat. Spray the pan with nonstick cooking spray, and then pour in the beaten eggs. Season with salt and pepper. Cook, stirring the eggs; when they just begin to form curds but are still quite wet, shake the pan to distribute them in an even layer and cook without stirring until the eggs still look a little wet on top, 3 to 4 minutes.

In a small skillet over medium heat, warm 2 tablespoons of the oil. Add the corn, red bell pepper, red onion, and green onion and cook, stirring, until soft, about 1 1/2 minutes. Add the crabmeat and corn mixture and cook until just heated through, about 2 minutes. Scrape the crabmeat mixture onto the center of the omelet. Fold the unfilled side over the filled side and transfer the omelet to a serving plate. Garnish with the fanned avocado slices and serve right away with the lemon wedge.

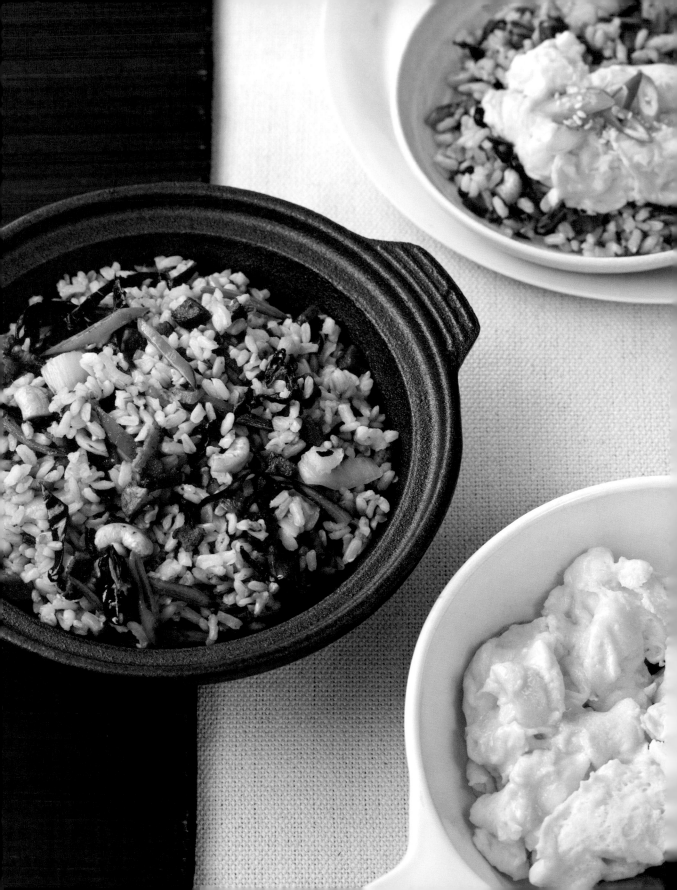

Breakfast Fried Rice with Scrambled Eggs

Think outside the (cereal) box: fried rice is a great way to fuel up with carbs in the morning. With brown rice, lots of fresh vegetables, and a minimal amount of fat, this recipe is a healthy take on fried rice and is high in vitamin B6. *Lop chong* is a dried, cooked Chinese sausage with a slightly sweet and smoky flavor; it will require a trip to the Asian grocery store, but you can choose to leave it out. MAKES 4 SERVINGS

FRIED RICE

2 tablespoons chopped lop chong (Chinese sausage; optional)

1/4 cup vegetable oil

1 tablespoon chopped garlic

1 tablespoon peeled, chopped fresh ginger

1 green onion, white and green parts, chopped

2 tablespoons diced red onion

2 tablespoons chopped fresh cilantro

1 or 2 leaves baby bok choy, thinly sliced

1/4 cup shredded red cabbage

5 sugar snap peas, cut into thin strips on the diagonal

2 cups cooked and cooled brown rice

4 tablespoons soy sauce

4 tablespoons mirin

EGGS AND GARNISHES

2 large eggs, beaten

1 teaspoon sesame seeds

2 tablespoons toasted cashews, chopped

1 green onion, white and green parts, sliced thin on the diagonal

To make the fried rice, in a large wok or large skillet over high heat, fry the *lop chong* until rendered, less than a minute. Transfer the *lop chong* to a paper towel–lined plate and discard the fat.

Set the wok over high heat and heat until very hot. Add the oil to the wok. Add the garlic, ginger, chopped green onion, red onion, cilantro, bok choy, cabbage, and snap peas. Cook, stirring, for 1 minute, or until the vegetables have softened and you can smell the ginger.

Add the rice and continue to cook, stirring, until everything is coated, 2 to 4 minutes. Add the soy sauce and mirin and toss well. Remove the wok from the heat.

To cook the eggs, heat a small nonstick skillet over medium heat. Spray the pan with nonstick cooking spray, and then pour in the beaten eggs. Cook, gently stirring the eggs for 1 to 2 minutes, until scrambled but still moist.

Transfer fried rice to a serving bowl and top with the scrambled eggs. Sprinkle with the sesame seeds, toasted cashews, and green onion and serve right away.

Asian Ratatouille Omelet

This omelet requires some time at the cutting board to prep the many vegetables and herbs, but cooking goes quickly and you'll be rewarded with an antioxidant-rich breakfast that's relatively low in saturated fat. **MAKES 1 OMELET, SERVING 1 OR 2**

4 tablespoons extra-virgin olive oil

1 tablespoon chopped garlic

1 tablespoon peeled, chopped fresh ginger

1/4 cup diced red or yellow bell pepper, or a mixture

2 tablespoons diced Japanese eggplant

2 tablespoons diced yellow summer squash

2 tablespoons diced zucchini

2 tablespoons diced red onion

2 tablespoons seeded, diced plum tomato

1 tablespoon chopped fresh basil leaves

4 large eggs, beaten

Salt and freshly ground black pepper

1 green onion, white and green parts, sliced thin on the diagonal

1/2 teaspoon sesame seeds

In a medium skillet over medium-high heat, warm the olive oil. Add the garlic and ginger and cook, stirring, until fragrant, about 20 seconds. Add the bell pepper, eggplant, squash, zucchini, red onion, tomato, and basil and cook until the vegetables are firm with a little golden color, about 4 minutes, stirring occasionally. Keep warm while cooking the eggs.

Heat a medium nonstick skillet over medium-high heat. Spray the pan with nonstick cooking spray, and then pour in the beaten eggs. Season with salt and pepper. Cook, stirring the eggs; when they just begin to form curds but are still quite wet, shake the pan to distribute them in an even layer and cook without stirring until there is just a little runny egg left, 3 to 4 minutes. It should still look a little wet on top. Add the vegetable filling perpendicular to the handle. By the time you've added the filling, the omelet will be set and you'll be ready to fold the omelet onto a plate. To plate, rest the lip of the pan almost in the center of the plate, tilt the plate and the pan against each other at a 45-degree angle, and then turn the pan over the plate quickly so that the omelet rolls off the pan and folds over onto the plate. Adjust with a fork if necessary. Garnish with the green onion and sesame seeds and serve right away.

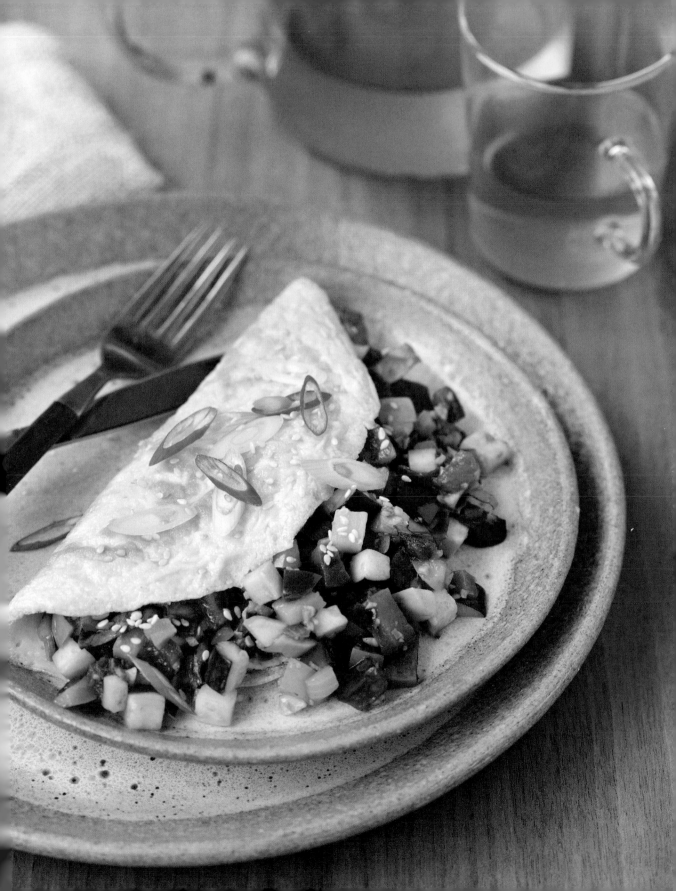

Gingered Spinach, Chicken, and Sun-Dried Tomato Omelet

This tasty omelet gets a protein boost from cooked chicken breast in the filling; it's a great way to turn leftovers from last night's roasted or grilled chicken into a healthy breakfast. Sun-dried tomatoes have a sweet, intense tomato flavor and add both vitamin C and vitamin A to the omelet. The spinach is high in polyphenol anti-oxidants, and even the basil garnish packs an antioxidant punch. MAKES 1 OMELET, SERVING 1 OR 2

2 tablespoons extra-virgin olive oil

1 teaspoon peeled, minced fresh ginger

1/4 cup diced cooked chicken breast

2 tablespoons chopped oil-packed sun-dried tomatoes

1/2 cup organic baby spinach

Salt and freshly ground black pepper

3 large eggs, beaten

In a medium skillet over medium heat, warm the oil. Add the ginger, chicken, and sun-dried tomatoes and cook, stirring occasionally, about a minute. Fold in the spinach and stir until it is wilted and the mixture is heated through, about 1 minute. Season to taste with salt and pepper. Keep warm while cooking the eggs.

Heat a medium nonstick skillet over medium-high heat. Spray the pan with nonstick cooking spray, and then pour in the beaten eggs. Season with salt and pepper. Cook, gently stirring the eggs; when they just begin to form curds but are still quite wet, shake the pan to distribute them in an even layer, and cook without stirring until the eggs still look a little wet on top, 3 to 4 minutes. Using a thin, wide spatula, flip the omelet and cook on the second side until the egg is cooked, about 1 minute. Remove the pan from the heat and scrape the chicken mixture over one half of the omelet. Fold the unfilled side over the filled side and transfer the omelet to a serving plate. Serve right away.

CHAPTER 10

Snacks and Starters

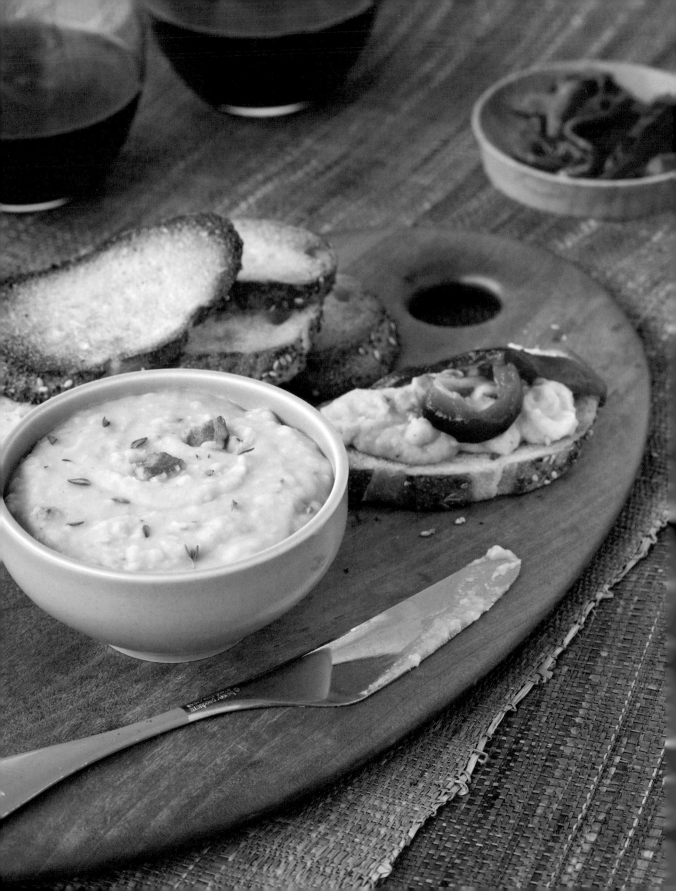

Cannellini Bean Dip with Roasted Red Peppers

This spread fits right in with the Mediterranean diet. Cannellini beans, a staple of Tuscany, Italy, are a great legume. Their benefit is further enhanced by the polyphenol-rich peppers and onions as well as the Brain-Boosting Broth. Try this dip on a piece of grilled artisan bread, with a little drizzle of extra-virgin olive oil.

MAKES ABOUT 2 CUPS

2 bacon slices, diced

2 tablespoons diced celery

2 tablespoons diced yellow onion

2 tablespoons peeled, diced parsnip

1 tablespoon chopped garlic

2 cups dried cannellini beans, soaked overnight and drained

5 cups Brain-Boosting Broth (page 130)

1 tablespoon chopped fresh thyme leaves

Salt and freshly ground black pepper

2 red bell peppers

In a large saucepan over medium heat, cook the bacon until the fat has rendered and the bacon is crisp, 4 to 6 minutes. Add the celery, onion, parsnip, and garlic and cook, stirring occasionally, until the vegetables begin to brown, about 2 minutes. Add the beans, broth, and thyme. Bring to a gentle simmer and cook, covered, until the beans are tender, 1 to 1^1/$_2$ hours.

With an immersion blender and using a pulsing action, puree the bean mixture in the pan, stopping when the dip has a nice, chunky texture. Season to taste with salt and pepper. Transfer to a serving bowl and let cool.

Roast the red bell peppers in the oven at 375°F on a baking sheet, on the grill, or held over a flame on a gas oven with tongs. Char the skin, rotating it for even charring, for 5 to 8 minutes. Once the skin starts cracking, place the peppers in a small bowl and cover the bowl with plastic wrap for 5 minutes. The skin will steep and separate from the peppers so that you can peel it off easily. Once the peppers are cool, peel and seed them, then cut into thin strips.

Arrange the red pepper strips on the dip and serve.

Herbed Pecans

This might be one of the simplest recipes in the book to prepare, but it's also one of the most delicious. Once you start eating these pecans, you simply cannot stop. The recipe was given to Chef Beau by Jan Weil, a guest who has visited Sanctuary for more than twenty-five years. At Jan's request, Beau made these nuts to serve at a charity event hosted by Jan at the resort. Pecans are a good source of vitamin E, and rosemary contains a very powerful antioxidant. **MAKES ABOUT 4 CUPS**

6 tablespoons unsalted butter
4 teaspoons dried rosemary
Generous pinch of salt
Pinch of cayenne pepper
Pinch of dried basil
4 cups pecan halves

Preheat the oven to 325°F.

In a large saucepan over medium heat, melt the butter. Add the rosemary, salt, cayenne, and basil and stir to combine. Remove the pan from the heat and add the pecans. Toss the pecans until they are well coated with the butter mixture, taking care not to break the nuts.

Distribute the pecans in an even layer on a rimmed baking sheet. Scrape any butter mixture remaining in the pan over the nuts. Bake for 10 to 12 minutes, or until well browned, gently stirring two or three times during baking.

Serve the pecans warm or at room temperature.

Crab Salad with Saffron

This recipe is an easy and fun start to a great brain-healthy meal with friends. The earthy, exotic flavor of the saffron is a nice match for the natural sweetness of the crab. The salad calls for only a small amount of saffron, but when used in a generous amount, the spice is a good source of riboflavin, folic acid, niacin, pyridoxine (one of the most important B vitamins for the brain), and vitamin C. The red bell pepper supplies color and crunch as well as polyphenol antioxidants, and the olive oil provides monounsaturated fat. Serve the salad over crisp rye chips—they're the perfect flavor and texture complement. **MAKES ABOUT 2 CUPS**

2 tablespoons low-fat or nonfat plain yogurt

Juice of 1 lemon

2 tablespoons extra-virgin olive oil

Pinch of saffron threads, crumbled

1 pound Dungeness or lump crabmeat

1 small yellow onion, finely diced

1/4 cup finely diced red bell pepper

Salt and freshly ground black pepper

Rye chips, for serving

1 tablespoon chopped fresh cilantro, for garnish

In a small nonreactive bowl, stir together the yogurt, lemon juice, olive oil, and saffron and let steep for at least 30 minutes.

Pick through the crabmeat, removing any shell and cartilage fragments. Break apart any large lumps with your fingers. Add the crabmeat to a medium bowl along with the onion, red bell pepper, and saffron mixture and fold to combine. Season to taste with salt and pepper. Top the rye chips with 1 tablespoon of the crab mixture and garnish each chip with cilantro before serving.

Roasted Eggplant Hummus

Beau has been serving this dish for years at Elements, his restaurant. The super-flavorful spread is an Asian balance of sweet, salty, spicy, sour, bitter, and savory tastes. It's also brain healthy in a few ways. Eggplant is a good source of polyphenol antioxidants, and olive oil is an excellent source of monounsaturated fat. The hummus is low in saturated fat and characteristic of the Mediterranean diet.

MAKES ABOUT 2 CUPS

2 to 3 Japanese eggplants (1 to 1¼ pounds)

2½ tablespoons soy sauce

1 teaspoon unseasoned rice vinegar

2½ tablespoons light brown sugar

2 tablespoons corn oil or peanut oil

1 tablespoon peeled, minced fresh ginger

1 tablespoon minced garlic

3 tablespoons minced green onions, white and green parts

½ teaspoon red pepper flakes

2 tablespoons toasted sesame oil

Salt and freshly ground black pepper

1 (15-ounce) can garbanzo beans, rinsed and drained

¼ cup tahini paste

1½ cups extra-virgin olive oil

Preheat the oven to 475°F.

Trim the top and bottom off each eggplant, rinse the eggplants, and pat dry. Prick each one with a fork in several places to create steam vents and set the eggplants on a rimmed baking sheet. Bake until the flesh gives easily when prodded, 20 to 40 minutes, depending on size; flip each eggplant midway through baking to ensure even cooking. When done, the eggplants will look like wrinkled, deflated balloons.

When cool enough to handle, slice open each eggplant along its length. Using a spoon, scoop the pulp from the skins and add it to a food processor. Discard the skins and the brown "liquor" that the eggplants may exude. Process the pulp until smooth. (Don't wash the food processor bowl; you'll need it to process the garbanzo beans.)

In a small bowl, combine the soy sauce, rice vinegar, and brown sugar. Stir until the sugar dissolves.

Heat a wok or large sauté pan over high heat and add the corn oil. Turn down the heat to medium-high and add the ginger, garlic, and green onions. Cook for a few seconds, stirring constantly, and then add the red pepper flakes. Continue to cook, stirring, until the mixture is fragrant, 20 to 40 seconds. Add the soy sauce mixture and cook until it boils around the edges of the wok, about 30 seconds. Add the eggplant pulp, stir well to combine, and cook until heated through, about 90 seconds. Turn off the heat and adjust the seasoning with salt and pepper. Stir in the sesame oil and set aside.

Combine the garbanzo beans and tahini in the food processor. With the machine running, slowly add the olive oil through the feed tube, until the hummus is creamy and smooth. Scrape down the bowl as needed. Transfer the garbanzo mixture to a bowl and stir in the eggplant mixture until combined. Adjust the seasoning with salt and pepper. Serve at room temperature. The hummus will keep in a sealed container in the refrigerator for 1 to 2 days.

Beet Hummus with Feta and Basil

In this recipe, roasted beet puree gives simple hummus a sweet, earthy flavor; a big jolt of color; and a dose of polyphenol antioxidants. The feta cheese garnish adds saltiness and acidity that contrasts with the taste of the spread, and the basil brings fresh, sweet herbal notes. If you have some basil pesto on hand, you can use it in place of the chopped basil. **MAKES ABOUT 2 CUPS**

BEET PUREE

2 large red beets, peeled and coarsely chopped

4 cups water

1 (15-ounce) can garbanzo beans, drained, with liquid reserved

1 cup Roasted Red Beet Puree (see above)

2 tablespoons freshly squeezed lemon juice

1 1/2 tablespoons tahini paste

2 teaspoons extra-virgin olive oil

2 cloves garlic, crushed

1 1/2 teaspoons salt

1/2 cup crumbled feta cheese

1/2 cup fresh basil leaves, chopped

To make the puree, combine the beets and water in a medium saucepan. Cover and bring to a boil over medium heat. Cook until the beets are soft, 10 to 15 minutes. Drain the beets, then place them in a blender or food processor and puree until smooth.

Combine the garbanzo beans and reserved liquid, beet puree, lemon juice, tahini, olive oil, garlic, and salt in a blender and puree until smooth, scraping down the sides of the jar as needed.

Transfer the hummus to a serving dish and garnish with the feta cheese and basil. Serve right away.

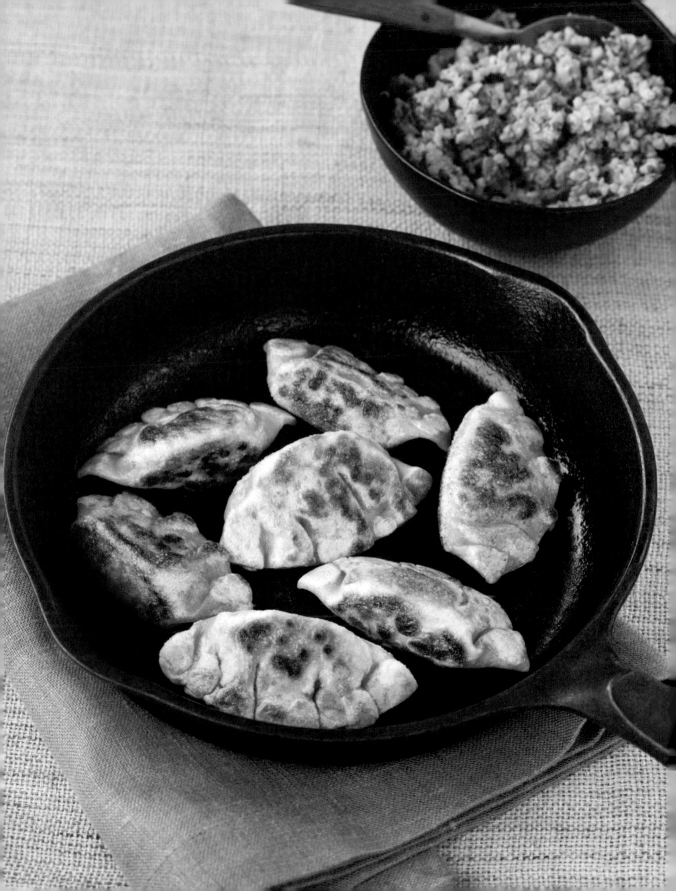

Sweet Potato and Quinoa Dumplings

Here is a recipe for tasty, healthful dumplings that are low in saturated fat. Quinoa is a very nutritious source of protein, and it makes a nice substitute for couscous with its nutty flavor. These dumplings integrate many healthy ingredients: anti-inflammatory ginger, antioxidant curry powder, and vitamin-rich sweet potatoes. Curry powder contains turmeric, a spice that may contribute to the reduced incidence of Alzheimer's disease in India. The dumpling dough takes some time and effort to make and roll out. You can use wonton or pot-sticker wrappers as a quick alternative, but you'll need to cut the wrappers into 2-inch circles with a cookie cutter before filling them. **MAKES ABOUT 32 DUMPLINGS, SERVING 8 TO 10**

DOUGH

2 cups all-purpose flour, plus more for dusting

1 cup boiling water

FILLING

1 sweet potato (about 8 ounces)

1 cup quinoa, rinsed and drained

2 cups water

2 teaspoons vegetable oil

1 teaspoon peeled, minced fresh ginger

1 teaspoon minced garlic

1 teaspoon curry powder

2 tablespoons chopped fresh cilantro leaves

1 teaspoon freshly squeezed lemon juice

1/4 cup low-fat or nonfat plain yogurt

Salt and freshly ground black pepper

Salt

Vegetable oil, for frying

Spicy Peanut Sauce (page 213) or Spinach Pesto Yogurt (page 211), for serving (optional)

To make the dough, place the flour in a large bowl. Slowly add the boiling water while stirring with a fork. Once all the water is incorporated, turn the dough out onto a lightly floured work surface. Dust your hands with some flour and knead by hand for about 3 minutes, or until the dough is worked into a firmer ball and the stickiness is gone. Keep adding flour to your hands to facilitate this process. Form the dough into a ball, wrap in plastic wrap, and refrigerate for 45 minutes.

Cut the dough ball in half. Working with one piece at a time, roll out each half on a lightly floured work surface into a sheet about 1/8 inch thick. Use a 2-inch round cookie cutter to cut out about 32 circles.

Preheat the oven to 325°F. To make the filling, pierce the skin of the sweet potato with a fork several times, then place in the oven on a baking sheet and roast for 45 minutes, or until soft. Let the sweet potato cool for 15 minutes in the refrigerator, peel the skin, and then finely chop the sweet potato.

To cook the quinoa, combine the quinoa and water in a medium saucepan and bring to a boil

continued

over high heat, reduce the heat to low, cover, and simmer until the water evaporates, about 15 minutes. Fluff with a fork.

In a large skillet over medium-high heat, warm the oil. Add the ginger and garlic, and cook, stirring, until fragrant, about 1 minute. Add the curry powder, cilantro, lemon juice, sweet potato, and quinoa and cook, stirring, just until the ingredients are well combined. Transfer to a medium bowl and stir in the yogurt. Season to taste with salt and pepper, cover, and refrigerate while preparing the dough.

To fill the dumplings, lay out a few dough circles on the work surface. Spoon about 2 tablespoons of filling onto each circle. Fold over into a half-moon shape, and pinch the edges with your fingers. If the edges aren't sticking, you can lightly brush the outsides of the circle with water before pinching together to bind the edges. Place the dumplings on a plate and cover with a damp towel to keep them from drying out before cooking (while you're forming the rest of the dumplings).

To cook the dumplings, bring a large pot of salted water to a boil over high heat. Add the dumplings in batches (8 to 10 at a time) and boil for 1 to 2 minutes. Remove the dumplings from the water with a slotted spoon. In a large nonstick skillet over medium heat, warm about 2 tablespoons of oil. Add as many dumplings as will comfortably fit in a single layer and cook until browned on all sides, about 30 seconds on each side, flipping them over so they evenly brown on both sides. Repeat to brown the remaining dumplings.

Serve immediately, either on their own or with Spicy Peanut Sauce or Spinach Pesto Yogurt.

Shrimp and Pork Pot Stickers

These pot stickers are a universal favorite at parties. Give yourself some time to get the folding right—Beau likes to fold his five times because five is a lucky number in China. **MAKES 36 TO 40 POT STICKERS**

3 tablespoons peanut oil

3 tablespoons peeled, minced ginger

3 tablespoons minced garlic

3 tablespoons minced fresh cilantro leaves

3 green onions, green and white parts, minced

1 pound shrimp, peeled, deveined, and finely chopped

1 pound ground pork

2 cups shredded napa cabbage

6 tablespoons toasted sesame oil

1 teaspoon salt

1 teaspoon freshly ground black pepper

1 package gyoza wrappers (about 50 wrappers)

1 large egg, beaten

About 2½ cups Brain-Boosting Broth (page 130) or water

Glaze (page 168), for serving

In a medium skillet over high heat, warm the peanut oil. Add the ginger, garlic, cilantro, and green onions and cook until fragrant, about 1 minute. Transfer to a medium bowl. Add the shrimp, pork, cabbage, sesame oil, salt, and pepper and mix well.

Dust a rimmed baking sheet with cornstarch to hold the filled pot stickers. Lay a few wrappers on a work surface; keep the rest covered to prevent them from drying out. Spoon a scant tablespoon of filling onto each wrapper and lightly brush the edges with beaten egg. Fold each wrapper in half to enclose the filling and form a half moon shape (if desired, pleat the edge of the top half of the wrapper as you bring the edges together); press to seal. Set the pot stickers on the prepared baking sheet and dust them with a little cornstarch to prevent sticking, and repeat until all of the filling is used.

Heat a nonstick skillet over medium-high heat. Spray the skillet with nonstick cooking spray and place as many pot stickers (pleated side up, if applicable) as will comfortably fit in a single layer; do not crowd the pan. Cook until the pot stickers are nicely browned, about 1 minute, and then add ½ cup broth. Cover and continue to cook until the liquid has evaporated, about 2 minutes. Take out one pot sticker and cut it in half to test for doneness. Transfer the pot stickers to a platter and serve or cover to keep warm while cooking subsequent batches. Serve with the Glaze as a dipping sauce.

Grilled Chicken Satay with Cucumber "Noodles," Yogurt-Mint Sauce, and Peanuts

Chicken satay is always a crowd-pleaser. In this version, coconut milk helps keep the chicken moist, while the antioxidant-rich turmeric in the curry powder helps keep your brain healthy. A refreshing yogurt sauce takes the place of the usual fat-laden peanut sauce, but tastes just as delicious. **MAKES 4 SERVINGS**

CHICKEN

2 (8-ounce) boneless, skinless chicken breasts
1 cup light coconut milk
1 teaspoon curry powder
1 teaspoon chopped garlic
1 tablespoon thinly sliced yellow onion
1 teaspoon smoked paprika
1 teaspoon red pepper flakes

CUCUMBER "NOODLES"

2 cucumbers
1 tablespoon chopped fresh mint leaves
1 tablespoon rice vinegar
Pinch of salt
Juice of 1 lime

YOGURT SAUCE

1 cup low-fat or nonfat plain yogurt
2 tablespoons chopped fresh mint leaves
Juice of 1 lime

1 cup roasted peanuts, chopped

Soak four 8- to 10-inch bamboo skewers in water to cover.

To marinate the chicken, using a sharp chef's knife, cut each chicken breast on the diagonal into thin strips. Thread the chicken strips onto the skewers and lay the skewers in a large baking dish. In a small bowl, mix the coconut milk, curry powder, garlic, onion, smoked paprika, and red pepper flakes. Pour this mixture over the chicken and turn the skewers to coat. Cover and refrigerate for at least 2 hours or up to 4 hours.

To prepare the "noodles," peel the cucumbers, cut it lengthwise in half, and scoop out the seeds. Cut each half into thin half-moons and add to a bowl along with the mint, vinegar, salt, and lime juice. Toss to coat, cover, and refrigerate for 1 hour.

To make the sauce, in a small bowl, mix the yogurt, mint, and lime juice. Refrigerate until needed.

To grill the chicken, build a hot fire in a charcoal grill or heat a gas grill on medium heat. Remove the chicken skewers from the marinade, wiping off any excess. When the grill is hot, cook the skewers until nicely browned on both sides, about 2 minutes.

To serve, place the cucumber "noodles" on a platter. Lay the skewers on top and sprinkle with the peanuts. Serve the sauce on the side.

Charred Shishito Pepper and Tomato Salsa

Dishes like this one that are high in vitamins and low in saturated fat are important for overall brain health. Both chiles and onions are good sources of polyphenols, and tomatoes provide vitamin E. If you can't find shishito peppers, you can use 2 Anaheim or 1 large poblano chiles. And if you can't find yuzu juice, just substitute freshly squeezed lemon or lime juice. This flavor-packed salsa can be served with tortilla chips as a snack or starter, and it goes great with scrambled egg whites.

MAKES ABOUT 1$\frac{1}{2}$ CUPS

1 cup shishito peppers, stemmed and cut into $\frac{1}{2}$-inch-thick rings

1$\frac{1}{2}$ teaspoons extra-virgin olive oil

Salt

2 large, ripe, semifirm heirloom tomatoes, diced

$\frac{1}{2}$ cup diced red onion

1 tablespoon jalapeño chiles, seeded and diced

1 tablespoon minced fresh cilantro leaves

1 tablespoon yuzu juice

Pinch of ground cumin, toasted

Pinch of red pepper flakes

Freshly ground black pepper

Position an oven rack in the upper third of the oven and preheat the broiler.

On a rimmed baking sheet, drizzle the shishito peppers with the oil, sprinkle with salt, and toss to combine. Distribute the peppers in an even layer and broil until nicely charred and caramelized, 2 to 3 minutes, turning them to char evenly halfway through roasting.

Dice the shishito peppers and transfer them to a nonreactive bowl. Add the tomatoes, onion, jalapeño, cilantro, yuzu juice, cumin, and red pepper flakes and toss to combine. Season to taste with salt and pepper. Serve right away.

Raw Oysters with Avocado, and Charred Shishito Pepper and Tomato Salsa

Beau is a big fan of oysters, and he thinks Island Creek oysters from Duxbury, Massachusetts, are some of the best on the planet. If you can find them, this recipe is a terrific way to serve them—the avocado and salsa really kick up their flavors. If you can't get Island Creek oysters, try Kumamoto or Wellfleet. Oysters are high in protein and low in saturated fat and cholesterol. They're also a good source for vitamins B and C. **MAKES 3 OR 4 SERVINGS**

12 fresh oysters, shucked, on the half shell, and chilled

1/3 cup Charred Shishito Pepper and Tomato Salsa (page 127)

1/2 ripe avocado, pitted, peeled, and diced small

Extra-virgin olive oil, for drizzling

Fill a large serving platter or tray with crushed ice. Set the oysters on the ice, making sure that they sit stably.

Spoon about 1 teaspoon of salsa on each oyster. Top each with a small spoonful of avocado, drizzle lightly with oil, and serve right away.

Avocado and Mango Salsa

This is a blue-chip recipe that can be served as a dip, as well as used in a variety of other ways. Its sweet, rich flavor is especially good with grilled fish and sautéed shrimp. Mangoes are full of flavonoids, and peppers are rich in vitamin C. **MAKES 2 1/2 CUPS**

1/4 serrano chile, seeded and minced

1 medium red bell pepper, seeded and diced medium

2 ripe mangoes, peeled and diced medium

2 1/2 tablespoons chopped fresh cilantro leaves

Juice of 2 limes

Salt

2 ripe avocados, pitted, peeled, and diced

Place the chile and bell pepper in a medium bowl and stir to combine. Add the mangoes and cilantro and mix gently. Season to taste with lime juice and salt. Gently fold in the avocados and adjust the seasoning with additional lime juice and salt. Serve right away or store in an airtight container in the refrigerator for up to 4 hours (any longer and the avocado will oxidize and turn brown).

Soups

Brain-Boosting Broth

This broth, the backbone of many of our soup recipes and an ingredient in many others, was developed with brain health in mind. It includes onions, fennel, parsley, oregano, and rosemary, all of which contain antioxidants, as well as parsnips, which are a good source of folic acid. The recipe uses water as the liquid, but you can start with chicken stock or fish stock to make an especially flavorful broth that would be great for sipping on its own. MAKES 2 QUARTS

8 quarts water

3 carrots, coarsely chopped

2 white onions, coarsely chopped

2 celery stalks, coarsely chopped

2 bulbs fennel, coarsely chopped

1 parsnip, coarsely chopped

12 cloves garlic, chopped

1/4 cup fresh ginger, peeled and chopped

Stems from 1/2 bunch fresh flat-leaf parsley

1 bunch green onions, green and white parts

1 stalk fresh lemongrass, cut in half lengthwise

1 tablespoon salt

1 teaspoon black peppercorns

2 cloves

1 teaspoon dried oregano

1 teaspoon dried rosemary

1 bay leaf

Combine all of the ingredients in a large stockpot and bring to a boil over high heat. Turn down the heat to maintain a gentle simmer and cook, uncovered, for 2 hours.

Strain the broth through a fine-mesh sieve. Use immediately, refrigerate for up to 5 days, or freeze for up to 1 month.

Chilled Beet Soup with Yuzu and Melon

This chilled soup is perfect for a hot summer day. It combines earthy beets, tangy yuzu juice (yuzu is a type of Japanese citrus), and sweet melons for a knockout flavor. But the soup doesn't just taste good; it's also beautiful to look at. And it gets even better: with plenty of polyphenol antioxidants from the beets and vitamin C from the melons and yuzu, the soup is excellent for brain health. If you can't find fresh yuzu, freshly squeezed lemon juice or lime juice will work as well.

MAKES 4 TO 6 SERVINGS

4 large red beets, trimmed

2 cucumbers, peeled, seeded, and coarsely chopped

1 medium shallot, coarsely chopped

1 medium cantaloupe, peeled, seeded, and chopped

1 medium honeydew, peeled, seeded, and chopped

1/4 cup yuzu juice

1 teaspoon ground coriander

1 cup low-fat or nonfat plain yogurt

Salt and freshly ground black pepper

Place the beets in a large pot of water and bring to a boil over medium-high heat. Boil the beets until a fork inserted into the largest beet meets no resistance, 15 to 20 minutes. Let cool to room temperature, and then slip off the skins. Cut the beets into chunks and add to a blender along with the cucumbers, shallot, cantaloupe, honeydew, yuzu juice, and coriander. Puree until smooth.

Strain the puree through a fine-mesh sieve into a bowl. Fold in the yogurt and season to taste with salt and pepper. Cover and refrigerate until well chilled, about 30 minutes to 1 hour.

Ladle the chilled soup into bowls and serve right away.

Curried Parsnip Soup

Sweet, earthy parsnips (which Beau likens to carrots on steroids) and spicy, fragrant curry powder are a tasty duo. This recipe yields a deliciously creamy soup that is low in saturated fat and that supports brain health with antioxidants in onion and the turmeric (turmeric is a key ingredient in curry powder), and monounsaturated fat in the olive oil. Parsnips are a great source of vitamin C and folic acid.

MAKES 6 TO 8 SERVINGS

2 tablespoons olive oil

1 pound parsnips, peeled and chopped

2 medium carrots, peeled and chopped

2 cloves garlic, chopped

1 medium white onion, chopped

2 tart apples, such as Granny Smith, peeled, cored, and chopped

1 teaspoon ground turmeric

2 tablespoons curry powder

1 jalapeño chile, seeded and chopped

2 1/2 quarts Brain-Boosting Broth (page 130)

1 cup nonfat milk

Salt and freshly ground black pepper

In a soup pot over medium-high heat, warm the olive oil. Add the parsnips, carrots, garlic, and onion, and cook, stirring, until softened, about 15 minutes. Add the apples, turmeric, curry, and jalapeño and cook, uncovered, until the apples soften, 3 to 4 minutes. Add the broth, increase the heat to high, and bring to a boil. Turn down the heat to maintain a simmer and cook until the parsnips and carrots are fully tender, 25 to 35 minutes.

Add the milk to the soup mixture. Working in batches if needed, puree the mixture in a blender until smooth. Return the soup to the pot and warm over medium heat until just heated through. Season to taste with salt and pepper, ladle into bowls, and serve.

Butternut Squash Soup with Miso

This soup is naturally sweet from the butternut squash and carrots; gets a subtle spicy, smoky kick from the chipotle chile; and salty, savory notes from the miso and soy sauce. Though its consistency is rich and creamy, the soup is low in saturated fat and supports brain health with a healthy dose of beta-carotene from the squash and carrots, as well as monounsaturated fat from the olive oil and polyphenol anti-oxidants from the onion. **MAKES 6 TO 8 SERVINGS**

2 butternut squashes (about 1 pound each)

3 tablespoons olive oil, plus more for coating the squash

2 medium carrots, peeled and chopped

1 medium white onion, chopped

6 cloves garlic, chopped

2 tablespoons peeled, minced fresh ginger

1 teaspoon sugar

1 teaspoon seeded, minced chipotle chile in adobo

2 quarts Brain-Boosting Broth (page 130)

1/4 cup low-sodium soy sauce

1/4 cup white miso

1 tablespoon rice vinegar

Preheat the oven to 300°F.

Cut each squash in half lengthwise and scoop out the seeds with a spoon. Pierce skin sides several times with fork and rub lightly with olive oil. Set the squash halves cut sides down on a rimmed baking sheet and roast until a fork inserted into the thickest part of the flesh meets no resistance, about 30 minutes. Let cool slightly.

Turn the squash halves cut sides up. Using a spoon, scoop the flesh from the skin and transfer to a bowl; discard the skins.

In a soup pot over medium heat, warm the olive oil. Add the carrots, onion, garlic, and ginger; cover; and cook, stirring occasionally, until the vegetables have begun to soften, about 15 minutes. Add the sugar, chile, and roasted squash and cook, stirring for 2 minutes. Add the broth, increase the heat to high, and bring to a boil. Turn down the heat to maintain a simmer and cook, uncovered, until the carrots are fully tender, 15 to 20 minutes. Stir in the soy sauce, miso, and vinegar.

Working in batches if needed, puree the mixture in a blender until smooth. Return the soup to the pot and warm over medium heat until just heated through. Ladle into bowls and serve.

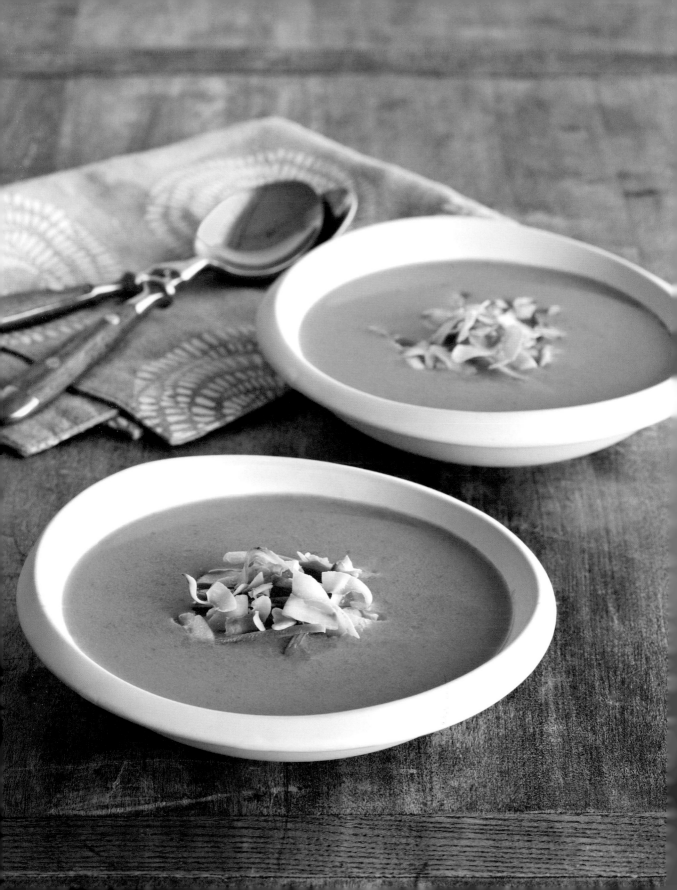

Carrot-Ginger Soup

Beau has been making this soup for more than fifteen years and it still surprises him how well carrots and ginger go together. This may be an everyday soup, but the addition of coconut milk adds silkiness and the kaffir lime leaves lend a surprising little zip. If you can't find kaffir lime leaves, the juice from 2 freshly squeezed limes can substitute. With polyphenol antioxidants from the bell peppers and onions as well as beta-carotene from the carrots, this soup is as good for you as it is delicious.

MAKES 6 TO 8 SERVINGS

1/4 cup vegetable oil

1 1/2 pounds carrots, peeled and chopped 1/2 inch thick

1 1/2 red bell peppers, seeded and chopped

2 medium yellow onions, chopped

1 sweet potato, peeled and chopped

1/4 cup peeled, chopped fresh ginger

Pinch of red pepper flakes

3 quarts Brain-Boosting Broth (page 130)

6 kaffir lime leaves

1 (15-ounce) can light coconut milk

1 teaspoon salt

Toasted coconut flakes, for garnish

In a soup pot over medium heat, warm the oil. Add the carrots, bell peppers, onions, sweet potato, red pepper flakes, and ginger; cover; and cook, stirring occasionally, until the vegetables have softened, about 15 minutes. Add the broth and kaffir leaves. Increase the heat to medium-high and bring to a boil, and then turn down to heat to maintain a soft rolling boil and cook, uncovered, for 45 minutes.

Add the coconut milk and salt. Remove and discard the kaffir leaves. Working in batches if needed, puree the soup in a blender until smooth. Return the soup to the pot and warm over medium heat until just heated through. Ladle into bowls, garnish with coconut, and serve.

Roasted Red Pepper Soup

Roasted red bell peppers give this soup an eye-catching color, a natural sweetness with hints of smokiness from the charred skins, and plenty of polyphenol antioxidants for brain health. The oregano adds distinctly Mediterranean flavor notes, and its extremely high ORAC score means that it provides potent antioxidants, too.

MAKES 4 TO 6 SERVINGS

8 red bell peppers

3 tablespoons oil

1 large yellow onion, chopped

3 cloves garlic, chopped

1½ teaspoons ground cumin

1 teaspoon dried oregano

1½ quarts Brain-Boosting Broth (page 130)

Salt and freshly ground black pepper

Roast the red bell peppers in the oven at 375°F on a baking sheet, on the grill, or held over a flame on a gas oven with tongs. Char the skin, rotating it for even charring, for 5 to 8 minutes. Once the skin starts cracking, place the peppers in a small bowl and cover the bowl with plastic wrap for 5 minutes. The skin will steep and separate from the peppers so that you can peel it off easily. Once the peppers are cool, peel and seed them, then coarsely chop.

In a soup pot over medium heat, warm the oil. Add the onion and garlic, cover, and cook, stirring occasionally, until the onion is translucent, 8 to 10 minutes. Add the roasted peppers and cook, stirring, until heated through, about 3 minutes. Stir in the cumin and oregano and cook until fragrant, about 1 minute. Pour in the broth, increase the heat to high, and bring to a boil. Turn down the heat to maintain a simmer and cook until the onion is fully softened and the flavors have blended, 15 to 20 minutes.

Working in batches if needed, puree the mixture in a blender until smooth. Return the soup to the pot and warm over medium heat until just heated through. Season to taste with salt and pepper, ladle into bowls, and serve.

Sweet Corn and Poblano Chile Soup

Sweet summer corn and mild, earthy poblano chiles are a terrific combination, especially when spiced up with cumin and chili powder as they are in this delicious soup. The potato thickens the soup so it has a nice consistency even without the addition of cream. Vitamin-rich vegetables and the nutritious Brain-Boosting Broth make this dish good for brain health. **MAKES 6 TO 8 SERVINGS**

2 poblano chiles

2 tablespoons vegetable oil

8 ears fresh sweet corn, shucked, kernels cut from cobs

2 medium yellow onions, chopped

1 leek, white and light green parts, chopped

1 celery stalk, chopped

8 cloves garlic, chopped

1 teaspoon chili powder

1 teaspoon ground cumin

3 bay leaves

1 medium potato, peeled and diced

3 quarts Brain-Boosting Broth (page 130)

Salt and freshly ground black pepper

Roast the chiles in the oven at 375°F on a baking sheet, on the grill, or held over a flame on a gas oven with tongs. Char the skin, rotating it for even charring, for 5 to 8 minutes. Once the skin starts cracking, place the chiles in a small bowl and cover the bowl with plastic wrap for 5 minutes. The skin will separate from the chiles so that you can peel it off easily. Once the chiles are cool, peel and seed them, then chop.

In a soup pot over medium heat, warm the oil. Add the corn, onions, leek, celery, and garlic; cover; and cook, stirring occasionally, until the vegetables have softened, 10 to 15 minutes. Add the poblano chiles, chili powder, cumin, and bay and cook, stirring, until the spices are well incorporated. Season with salt, add the potato, and pour in the broth. Increase the heat to high, bring to a boil, and then turn down the heat to maintain a simmer. Cook until the vegetables are fully tender, about 25 minutes.

Working in batches if needed, puree the mixture in a blender until smooth. Strain the puree through a fine-mesh sieve and return the soup to the pot. Warm over medium heat until just heated through and season to taste with salt and pepper. Ladle into bowls and serve.

Brain-Boosting Buckwheat Noodle Bowl

This recipe is food for the soul. It's a warm, delicious, flavorful broth that incorporates ginger, miso, and light soy sauce, as well as healthy vegetables, and buckwheat—also called soba—noodles. Consider this an everyday eat or for whenever you need a little brain boost. And, it's a great building-block recipe to add to your repertoire because you can do a lot to it—add some chili paste, shredded chicken, or shrimp—to make it your own. **SERVES 2**

$2^{1}/_{2}$ cups Brain-Boosting Broth (page 130)

1 teaspoon peeled, grated fresh ginger

1 tablespoon miso

2 tablespoons low-sodium soy sauce

4 ounces soba noodles

2 fresh shiitake mushrooms, sliced

6 fresh whole beach mushrooms, ends of stems trimmed

2 kale leaves, chopped

$^{1}/_{8}$ yellow bell pepper, sliced

$^{1}/_{4}$ cup sliced carrots

1 baby bok choy, sliced

2 green onions, green parts only, sliced on the diagonal, for garnish

In a soup pot over medium-high heat, bring the broth to a boil. Add the ginger, miso, and soy sauce, then lower heat to medium and let simmer for 5 minutes.

Fill a medium pot two-thirds full with water and bring to a boil over high heat. Add the soba noodles and cook until al dente, about 1 or 2 minutes. Keeping the water boiling, use a slotted spoon to remove the cooked noodles from the pot and transfer to a colander. When cool, transfer the noodles to a large serving bowl.

Add the shiitake mushrooms, beach mushrooms, kale, bell pepper, carrot, and bok choy to the pot of boiling water for less than 1 minute. Drain.

Arrange the vegetable mixture over the noodles, then pour in the broth. Garnish with green onions and serve.

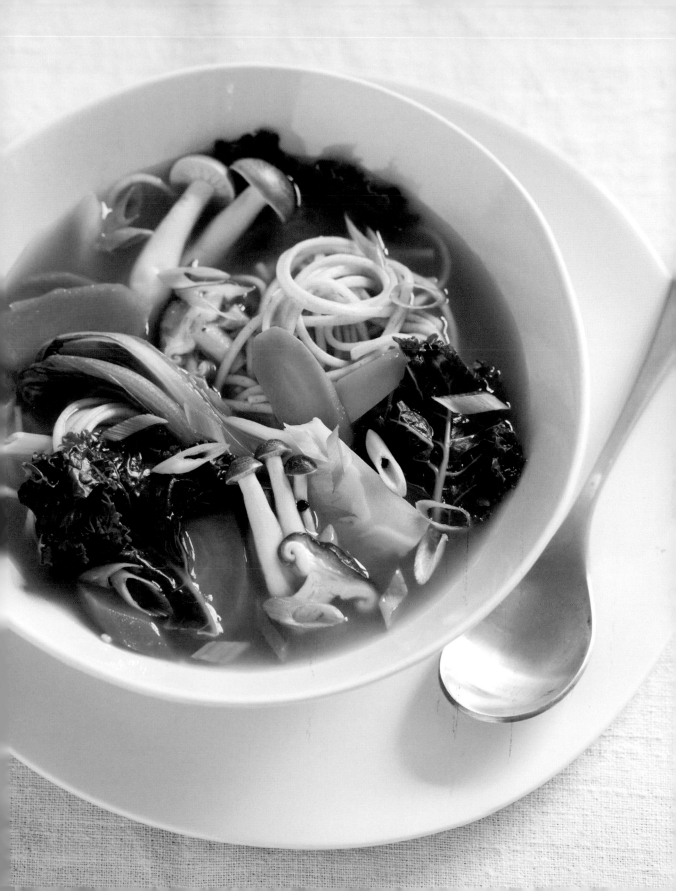

Strawberry-Cinnamon Soup with Herbed Pecans

This chilled soup can be served as a first course or as the conclusion to a meal. If you're serving it as dessert, a scoop of mango or pineapple sorbet in each bowl is a great addition. Make this recipe when strawberries are in season and flavorful; if they're on the tart side, don't be afraid to compensate with a little honey if you need to. With fresh strawberries, ground cinnamon, and oregano, this recipe is rich in antioxidants for good brain health. **MAKES 4 TO 6 SERVINGS**

2 pints fresh, ripe strawberries, hulled and chopped

2 cups orange juice

2 cups Brain-Boosting Broth (page 130), chilled

1 cup honey

Pinch of fresh basil

Pinch of fresh oregano

1 tablespoon ground cinnamon

8 fresh mint leaves

Pinch of salt

Pinch of freshly ground black pepper

$1/2$ cup Herbed Pecans (page 118), for garnish

To make the soup, combine the strawberries, orange juice, broth, honey, basil, oregano, cinnamon, mint, salt, and pepper and let sit in the refrigerator for 1 to 2 hours. Pour the mixture into a blender and puree until smooth. Strain through a fine-mesh sieve into a bowl. Sweeten to taste with honey as needed. Let the soup chill in the refrigerator for about an hour before serving.

To serve, ladle the soup into bowls and garnish with a sprinkling of pecans.

CHAPTER 12

Salads and Sandwiches

Warm Spinach Salad with Oranges and Sunflower Seeds

Spinach is usually what comes to mind when the doctor recommends a diet featuring plenty of leafy green vegetables. There's a good reason for this: spinach is one of the most antioxidant-rich vegetables out there. In this salad, the oranges add bright color and flavor, as well as a good dose of vitamin C, and the sunflower seeds offer a pleasing crunch and vitamin E as a bonus. By adding a piece of seared salmon, you can turn this salad into a main-dish meal. MAKES 4 SERVINGS

SPINACH SALAD

10 oranges

1 pound fresh shiitake
mushrooms, stemmed and
very thinly sliced

13 cups baby spinach

MUSTARD DRESSING

1/4 cup sugar

1 teaspoon mustard powder
(such as Coleman's)

2 egg yolks

1/4 cup red wine vinegar

Salt and freshly ground black
pepper

1/2 cup shelled sunflower
seeds, toasted

To make the salad, cut off the top and bottom of each orange and set the fruit on a cut end. Working from top to bottom and following the contour of the orange, use a sharp knife to trim away the peel with the pith in strips, rotating the fruit after each cut. Hold the fruit in your hand and make a pole-to-pole cut between the membrane and the flesh of each section to free the orange segments. Add the segments to a large bowl, along with the mushrooms and spinach.

To make the dressing, combine the sugar and mustard in a stainless-steel bowl and mix over a pot of simmering water, being careful not to overheat, until the sugar dissolves, about 30 seconds to a minute. Combine the egg yolks and vinegar in a separate bowl and then mix the two mixtures together in the bowl over the water. Continue cooking the mustard mixture in the double-boiler, whisking vigorously and continuously over a low simmer for 4 to 8 minutes, until it is incorporated, the graininess of the mustard disappears, and the mixture thickens and expands. Remove from heat.

Drizzle the warm dressing over the spinach mixture and toss gently until evenly coated. Season to taste with salt and pepper. Divide the salad among serving plates, garnish with the sunflower seeds, and serve right away.

Avocado, Tomato, and Red Onion Salad

The key to this salad is the produce: make sure to use avocados that are perfectly ripe, as well as in-season, garden-fresh tomatoes. High-quality olive oil wouldn't hurt, either. Beau believes that parsley is an underutilized, underrated herb; here, a generous amount of fresh parsley adds a nice little grassy sharpness to the flavor profile. Though the salad is rich in taste and texture thanks to the avocado, it is very low in saturated fat. The onion and parsley add an antioxidant boost to help support brain health. **MAKES 3 TO 4 SERVINGS**

1 pound ripe heirloom tomatoes, cored and coarsely chopped

Sea salt

Freshly ground black pepper

2 large ripe avocados, halved

1/2 cup thinly sliced red onion

1 cup flat-leaf parsley leaves

1 tablespoon extra-virgin olive oil

Juice of 1 lemon

Arrange the tomato pieces on a platter and season with salt and pepper.

Pit, peel, and cut each avocado half into rough cubes. Add the avocado cubes to a medium bowl along with the onion and parsley. Drizzle with the olive oil and lemon juice and toss gently to combine.

Place the avocado mixture on top of the tomatoes. Season to taste with salt and pepper and serve right away.

Arugula and Fennel Salad with Pomegranate Vinaigrette

In this salad full of clean, fresh flavors, all the ingredients really shine. Fennel is a very good source of vitamin C. When pomegranates are in season—October through January is typically when they are at their best—a garnish of sprinkled pomegranate seeds over the salad adds an antioxidant boost. **MAKES 6 SERVINGS**

2 tablespoons champagne vinegar

4 tablespoons pomegranate juice

1/2 cup extra-virgin olive oil

Salt and freshly ground black pepper

3 oranges

1 fennel bulb, shaved

13 cups baby arugula

1/2 cup Herbed Pecans (page 118)

Pour the vinegar into a medium bowl and add the pomegranate juice. Gradually whisk in the olive oil. Season to taste with salt and pepper.

Cut off the top and bottom of the oranges and set the fruit on a cut end. Working from top to bottom and following the contour of the orange, use a sharp knife to trim away the peel with the pith in strips, rotating the fruit after each cut. Hold the fruit in your hand and make a pole-to-pole cut between the membrane and the flesh of each section to free the orange segments.

In a large bowl, combine the fennel, oranges, and arugula. Drizzle with the dressing, sprinkle with the pecans, and toss gently. Season to taste with salt and pepper and serve right away.

Tomato and Arugula Salad with Parmigiano-Reggiano

Arugula is a leafy green vegetable that is commonly used in Italian cooking. It is a good source of phytonutrients as well as of vitamins A, B, and C. In this salad, arugula's pleasantly bitter, peppery flavor is balanced by the sweetness of the tomatoes and balsamic vinegar and by the nutty savoriness of the Parmesan cheese. Because there are so few ingredients in this simple recipe, quality really counts, so be sure to use the best-quality produce, olive oil, and cheese that you can get your hands on. **MAKES 4 TO 6 SERVINGS**

$3/4$ pound ripe tomatoes

Salt and freshly ground black pepper

13 cups baby arugula

1 large red onion, chopped

$1/4$ cup extra-virgin olive oil

3 tablespoons balsamic vinegar

3 ounces Parmigiano-Reggiano cheese

Core the tomatoes and chop them coarsely. Season with salt and pepper.

Place the arugula in a large serving bowl and top with the tomatoes and onion. Drizzle with the olive oil and balsamic vinegar and season to taste with salt and pepper. Using a vegetable peeler, shave the cheese over the salad, then toss gently and serve right away.

Arugula, Jicama, and Roasted Corn Salad

In this salad, the peppery bite of the arugula; the sweetness of the jicama, corn, and tomatoes; and the zestiness of the dressing work together perfectly. And with the jicama's crunch and the corn's crispness, the salad has a terrific texture to match its great taste. The olive oil in the dressing supplies monounsaturated fat, and the variety of vegetables means you benefit from multiple sources of vitamins, with the arugula offering a wealth of phytonutrients. MAKES 4 SERVINGS

4 ears fresh corn, unshucked

1/2 cup extra-virgin olive oil

3 tablespoons freshly squeezed orange juice

1 tablespoon champagne vinegar

1 teaspoon minced shallot

1 teaspoon honey

1/2 teaspoon Dijon mustard

1/2 teaspoon grated lemon zest or lime zest

1/2 teaspoon freshly ground black pepper

1/4 teaspoon salt, plus more to taste

13 cups baby arugula

8 ounces jicama, peeled and cut into matchsticks (about 1 cup)

2 cups cherry tomatoes, preferably heirloom, halved

4 teaspoons chopped fresh cilantro leaves

Soak the ears of corn in a pot of water for 3 hours. If roasting on the grill, roast in the husk over medium heat, turning regularly, for about 15 minutes. You can also roast the corn in the husk in a 325°F oven for 25 minutes, turning the husks regularly. Remove the ears of corn from the heat and leave in husk to finish cooking. Let cool for about 30 minutes, then shuck the corn husks and trim the corn kernels off the cob using a knife and slicing down the ear vertically.

In a medium bowl, whisk together the olive oil, orange juice, vinegar, shallot, honey, mustard, lemon zest, pepper, and 1/4 teaspoon salt.

Combine the corn, arugula, jicama, tomatoes, and cilantro in a large bowl. Pour the dressing over and toss gently. Transfer to a serving platter and season to taste with salt. Serve right away.

Grilled Corn, Edamame, and Tomato Salad

Edamame is one of Beau's favorite snacks. Not only do the shelled beans taste great, but with lots of fiber and vitamins, they're great for you, too. Mix edamame with corn, tomatoes, and red bell pepper, and you get this flavorful, festive-looking salad that can double as a condiment for grilled seafood. Fresh chervil, an herb that contains in B vitamins, is sometimes called "French parsley"; if it's unavailable, you can substitute regular parsley. **MAKES 4 SERVINGS**

2 ears fresh corn, unshucked

1 pound cherry or cocktail tomatoes, cored and quartered

1 red bell pepper, seeded and diced small

2 green onions, white and green parts, chopped

2 cups shelled, cooked edamame

1 teaspoon truffle oil

2 tablespoons rice wine vinegar

2 tablespoons extra-virgin olive oil

1 teaspoon smoked paprika

1 head of butter lettuce, quartered

Salt and freshly ground black pepper

1 bunch fresh chervil, leaves chopped

Put the ears of corn in a bowl and add warm water to cover. Let soak for 30 minutes.

Build a cool fire in a charcoal grill or heat a gas grill on low heat. Remove the corn from the water and grill the ears in their husks until the kernels are tender, about 15 minutes. Shuck the corn, cut the kernels from the cobs, and add to a large bowl along with the tomatoes. Toss to combine. Add the red bell pepper, green onions, edamame, truffle oil, vinegar, and olive oil and toss again. Place quartered lettuce on four plates and spoon over the salad mixture. Season to taste with salt and pepper, sprinkle with the chervil, and serve right away.

Kale, Blueberry, and Pomegranate Salad

Kale is usually thought of as a green for cooking, but in this recipe, it's used as a salad green, one with a lot more texture than lettuce. Its hardiness means that the leaves won't wilt after the salad is dressed. Kale's pleasant bitterness is nicely balanced by the sweetness of the blueberries and the tartness of the pomegranate seeds. This salad is rich in brain-boosting foods: kale is an excellent source of flavonoids and vitamin C, blueberries are high in antioxidants, and pomegranates provide a great source of resveratrol. **MAKES 4 SERVINGS**

3 bunches kale, stemmed and chopped

1 cup fresh blueberries

2 medium carrots, peeled and shredded

1/2 cup pomegranate seeds

1/3 cup pumpkin seeds, toasted

1/3 cup sliced almonds, toasted

1 tablespoon chopped fresh mint leaves

1/2 cup Soy-Sesame Vinaigrette (page 210)

Salt and freshly ground black pepper

Combine the kale, blueberries, carrots, pomegranate seeds, pumpkin seeds, almonds, and mint in a medium bowl and toss well. Drizzle with the vinaigrette and toss again. Season to taste with salt and pepper and serve right away.

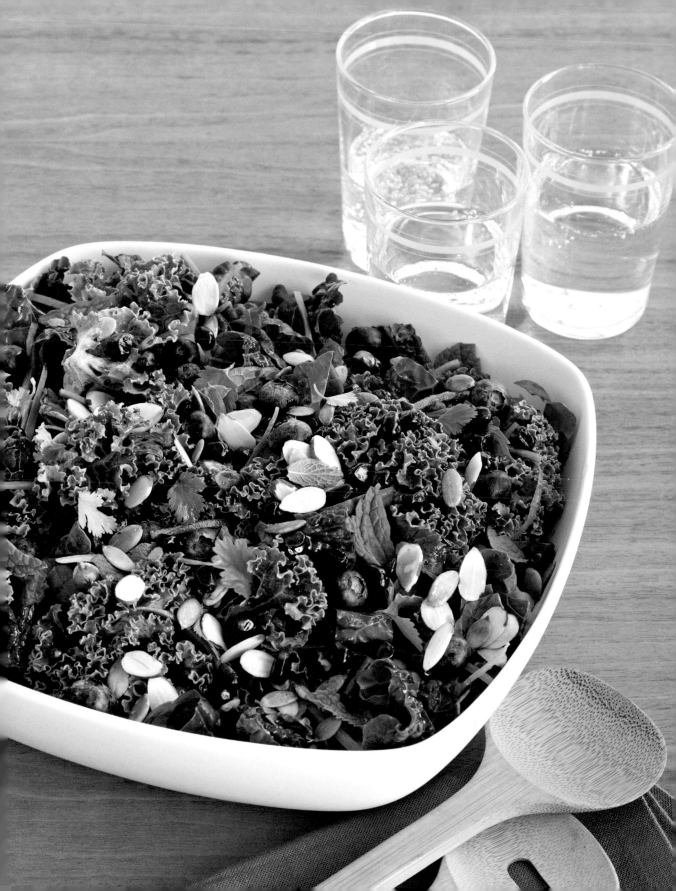

Watercress and Avocado Salad with Grapefruit

Watercress adds a hint of pepperiness to this easy-to-prepare salad. If you don't want to use grapefruit (an excellent source of vitamin C), ripe mango sections also work well, but you will have tropical, sweet notes in the salad instead of the tart bitterness of the grapefruit. Aside from being delicious, avocados are rich in folic acid and vitamin B6. **MAKES 4 TO 6 SERVINGS**

6 grapefruits

1/2 cup extra-virgin olive oil

1 tablespoon honey

1 tablespoon shredded fresh basil leaves, plus 1/4 cup torn fresh basil leaves, for garnish

1 teaspoon minced shallot

1/2 teaspoon Dijon mustard

1/4 teaspoon minced garlic

Salt and freshly ground black pepper

3 large ripe avocados, pitted, peeled, and sliced into eighths

6 bunches organic watercress, stemmed to leave 2 inches of stem (about 9 cups)

1/2 cup torn fresh mint leaves, for garnish

Cut off the top and bottom of the grapefruits and set the fruit on a cut end. Working from top to bottom and following the contour of the grapefruit, use a sharp knife to trim away the peel with the pith in strips, rotating the fruit after each cut. Hold the fruit in your hand and make a pole-to-pole cut between the membrane and the flesh of each section to free the grapefruit segments.

In a large bowl, combine the grapefruits, olive oil, honey, shredded basil, shallot, mustard, and garlic. Season to taste with salt and pepper.

Add the avocado slices to the dressing mixture and toss so that every slice gets coated with the dressing. Add the watercress to the avocado and dressing mixture and gently fold to incorporate. Transfer to a serving platter and garnish with the torn basil and mint. Serve right away.

Hearts of Palm Salad with Cucumber and Zucchini

This recipe brings together a handful of brain-healthy elements to create a hearty, chunky salad that's low in saturated fat. The hearts of palm are a good source of vitamin C, and the onion supplies polyphenol antioxidants. Both the parsley and cumin contain antioxidants, too, and the olive oil adds healthy monounsaturated fat. If it's at all possible, purchase fresh hearts of palm (check Asian markets if you can't find them in your regular store). The canned version pales in comparison, so use it only if you have no other choice. If you can't find yuzu juice, substitute lemon or lime juice. MAKES 4 SERVINGS

4 ounces fresh hearts of palm, sliced into 1/4-inch rounds (about 2 cups)

1 English cucumber, peeled and sliced 1/4 inch thick

1 medium zucchini, peeled and sliced 1/4 inch thick

1 ripe heirloom tomato, cored, quartered, and sliced

1 yellow onion, very thinly sliced

1 cup fresh flat-leaf parsley leaves, plus 4 flat-leaf parsley leaves, for garnish

2 tablespoons extra-virgin olive oil, plus more for drizzling

2 tablespoons yuzu juice

1 tablespoon paprika

1 teaspoon ground cumin

Salt and freshly ground black pepper

Combine the hearts of palm, cucumber, zucchini, tomato, onion, 1 cup of parsley leaves, olive oil, yuzu juice, paprika, and cumin in a large bowl. Toss to combine, cover, and refrigerate for 15 minutes to allow the flavors to blend.

Let stand at room temperature for 15 minutes before serving. When ready to serve, season to taste with salt and pepper, drizzle with olive oil, and garnish with the remaining parsley leaves.

Roasted Beet Salad with Arugula, Frisée, and Balsamic Glaze

There are lots of big flavors working in this dish. The recipe takes some time to prepare, but the reward in the end is a beautiful and tasty salad that will impress your guests. And since beets are rich in polyphenol antioxidants, the salad will also help keep your guests' brains healthy. If you can, use beets of different colors—red, golden, and even striped beets are sold in grocery stores and farmers' markets these days. **MAKES 4 SERVINGS**

BALSAMIC GLAZE

1 tablespoon olive oil
3/4 teaspoon chopped garlic
3/4 teaspoon minced shallot
Pinch of red pepper flakes
1 sprig thyme
2 cups balsamic vinegar
1 cup honey

SALAD

6 medium beets, trimmed
Olive oil, for roasting
2 tablespoons crème fraîche
Zest from 1 large lemon
1 bunch chives, chopped
Salt and freshly ground black pepper
4 cups loosely packed arugula
2 heads frisée, leaves separated
1/2 cup loosely packed torn fresh basil leaves

To make the glaze, in a small nonreactive saucepan over medium heat, warm the oil. Add the garlic, shallot, red pepper flakes, and thyme and cook, stirring, until the shallot softens, less than a minute. Pour in the vinegar, bring to a simmer, and cook until reduced to 1 cup, about 60 minutes. Remove from the heat and let cool, then add the honey and cook for 5 minutes, stirring to incorporate. Strain the mixture through a very fine mesh strainer into an airtight container and let cool.

To make the salad, preheat the oven to 370°F.

Lightly brush the beets with oil, wrap them in aluminum foil, and bake until a fork inserted into the center meets no resistance, 45 to 60 minutes. Unwrap and let cool.

Slip the skins off the beets. Cut each beet into quarters and add to a medium bowl. Add the crème fraîche, lemon zest, and chives and toss to combine. Season to taste with salt and pepper.

Divide the arugula, frisée, and basil leaves among four plates. Drizzle each plate with 1 tablespoon of the balsamic glaze, toss gently, and serve right away. (Leftover glaze can be stored in an airtight container in the refrigerator for up to 1 month.)

Beet and Melon Salad with Mixed Berries

Earthy beets are a nice contrast to musky cantaloupe and tart berries. You can serve this salad "sweet" on top of a bowl of Greek-style yogurt or you can mix in some chopped fresh kale and have it as a savory dish. The recipe delivers a double whammy of polyphenol antioxidants from the beets and the berries; the latter are among the brain-healthiest fruits you can find. If you can't find yuzu juice, substitute lemon or lime juice. MAKES 3 OR 4 SERVINGS

20 baby beets, trimmed

Extra-virgin olive oil, for roasting

Salt

1 cup peeled, seeded, and diced cantaloupe

1/2 cup mixed fresh berries (blueberries, raspberries, and blackberries)

1 tablespoon shredded fresh mint leaves

1 tablespoon honey

Juice of 1 lemon

1 teaspoon yuzu juice

Preheat the oven to 350°F.

Place the beets in an ovenproof pan and toss them with a little oil and salt. Wrap the beets in aluminum foil and bake until a fork inserted into the center meets no resistance, 15 to 20 minutes. Unwrap and let cool.

Slip the skins off the beets. Cut each beet in half and add to a medium bowl along with the cantaloupe, berries, mint, honey, lemon juice, and yuzu juice. Toss gently to combine. Serve right away.

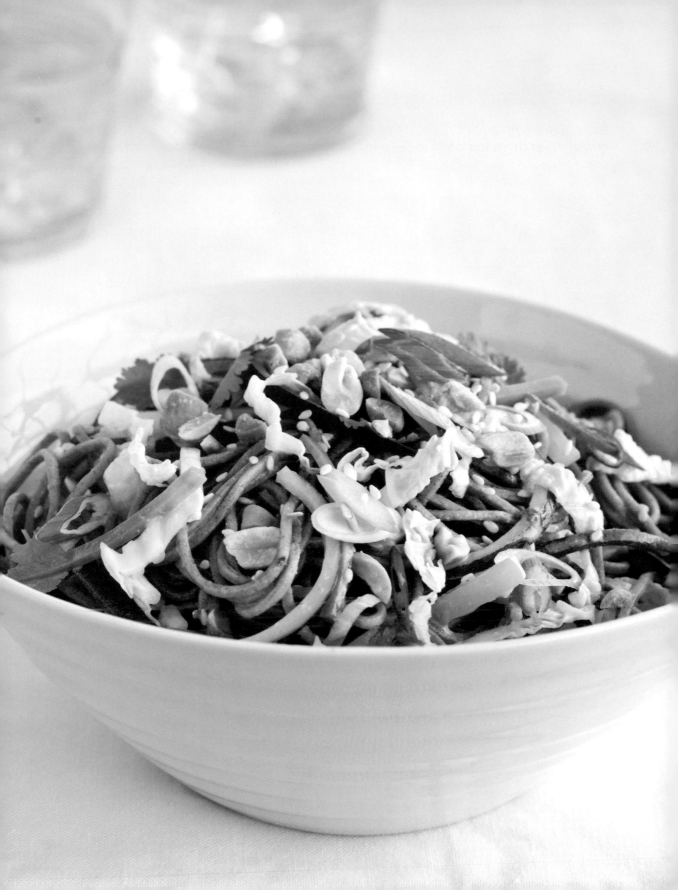

Soba Noodle Salad with Spicy Peanut Sauce

You might be tempted to rinse the noodles under running water after cooking and draining them, but don't. Beau prefers to leave starch clinging to the noodles because it picks up the dressing better. However, make sure to toss the cooked and drained noodles with oil so that the strands won't stick together. This dish is very flavorful and satisfying, yet is low in saturated fat. The onion and peppers add vibrant color and crunch to the salad, as well as polyphenol antioxidants that support brain health. You can serve the noodles at room temperature or chilled.

MAKES 4 SERVINGS

1 pound soba noodles

2 tablespoons extra-virgin olive oil

1 cup shredded napa cabbage

1/4 cup thinly sliced red onion

1 large red bell pepper, seeded and cut into matchsticks

1 large yellow bell pepper, seeded and cut into matchsticks

1 large carrot, peeled and cut into matchsticks

1/4 cup fresh cilantro leaves

1 cup Spicy Peanut Sauce (page 213)

3/4 cup roasted peanuts, coarsely chopped

4 green onions, sliced thin on the diagonal

1 tablespoon sesame seeds

Fill a large pot two-thirds full with water and bring to a boil over high heat. Add the noodles and cook until al dente. Drain in a colander (don't rinse them under running water) and transfer to a large bowl. Drizzle with the olive oil and toss gently until the noodles are coated. Let the noodles cool to room temperature.

Add the cabbage, red onion, red bell pepper, yellow bell pepper, carrot, and cilantro to the noodles and toss to combine. Pour the peanut sauce over and toss again until the noodles and vegetables are evenly coated with sauce.

Transfer to a serving bowl; garnish with the peanuts, green onions, and sesame seeds; and serve.

Ahi Tuna on Rye with Spinach Pesto Yogurt

This is not your average tuna sandwich. For one thing, it's more like tuna tartare on bread. For another, it's a very brain-healthy meal. Spinach Pesto Yogurt (page 211), not mayonnaise, holds the tuna mixture together, which keeps the amount of saturated fat to a minimum. Tuna is an excellent source of omega-3 fatty acids, the pistachios provide vitamin E, and the raisins are a good source of polyphenol antioxidants. Because the tuna is not cooked in this recipe, be sure to purchase sashimi-grade tuna; ask the fishmonger if you aren't sure about the quality of the tuna on offer at the seafood counter. MAKES 2 SANDWICHES

8 ounces sashimi-grade ahi tuna, diced small

2 tablespoons Spinach Pesto Yogurt (page 211)

2 tablespoons golden raisins

$1/4$ cup shelled unsalted roasted pistachios, chopped

Juice of $1/2$ lemon

4 slices rye bread, toasted

$1/2$ cup alfalfa sprouts

1 teaspoon extra-virgin olive oil

In a medium bowl, combine the tuna, Spinach Pesto Yogurt, raisins, pistachios, and lemon juice, and mix well.

Lay out two of the bread slices on a work surface and divide the tuna mixture evenly among them. Put the alfalfa sprouts into a small bowl, drizzle with the olive oil, and toss to combine. Top each portion of tuna with half of the alfalfa sprouts and top with the remaining slices of bread. Cut each sandwich in half and serve right away.

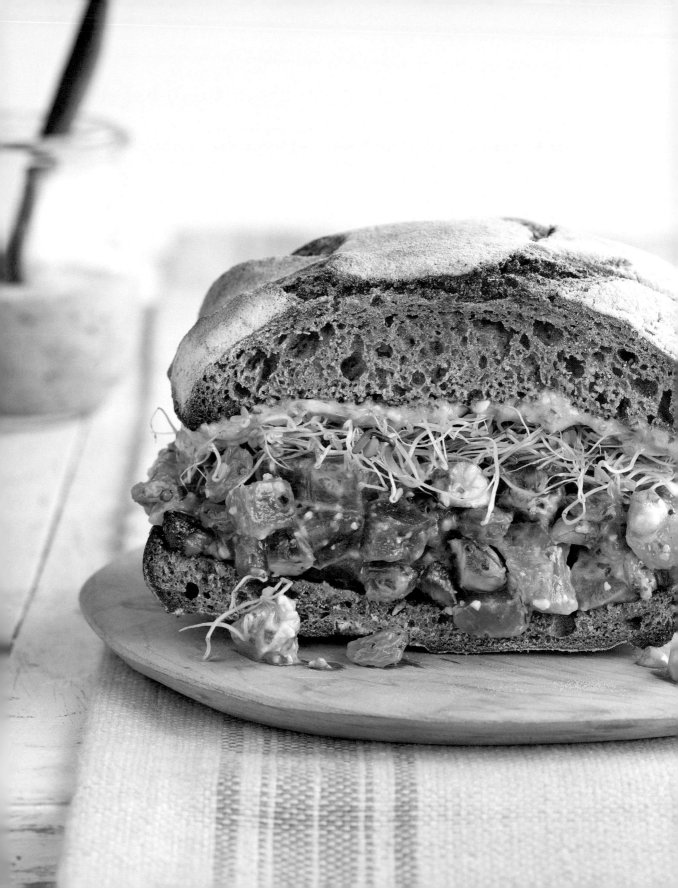

Turkey on 9-Grain with Black Bean Salsa and Tarragon Yogurt

Roasted turkey breast is a healthy and tasty source of protein, but these sandwiches are equally good with grilled chicken breast or lean roast beef instead. The black bean salsa, made with fresh tomato and green onion, brings a delicious savoriness to the mix as well as brain-healthy vitamin B6 (from the beans), vitamin E (from the sunflower seeds), and antioxidants (from the cumin). And add to that the antioxidants from the tarragon and the fiber from the whole-grain bread . . . these are sandwiches are powerhouses of good nutrition. MAKES 2 SANDWICHES

BLACK BEAN SALSA

1/2 cup rinsed and drained canned black beans

1 small ripe tomato, seeded and chopped

1 tablespoon green onion, sliced thin

1 tablespoon shelled sunflower seeds, toasted

1/2 teaspoon ground cumin

1/2 teaspoon paprika

Salt

Freshly squeezed lemon juice

TARRAGON YOGURT

1/2 cup low-fat or nonfat plain yogurt

1 sprig tarragon, chopped

Freshly squeezed lemon juice

Salt and freshly ground black pepper

4 slices 9-grain or other multigrain bread, toasted

10 ounces sliced roasted turkey breast

1/2 cup alfalfa sprouts

To make the salsa, in a small bowl, stir together the beans, tomato, green onion, sunflower seeds, cumin, and paprika. Season to taste with salt and lemon juice.

To make the yogurt, in a second small bowl, stir together the yogurt and tarragon. Season to taste with salt, pepper, and lemon juice.

To assemble the sandwiches, lay out the bread slices on a work surface and spread about 2 tablespoons of the yogurt mixture on one side of each slice. Arrange the turkey on 2 of the slices, dividing it evenly. Spoon salsa onto the turkey, and then top with the sprouts. Place the remaining bread slices, yogurt side down, on top. Cut each sandwich in half and serve right away.

CHAPTER 13

Main Dishes

Soba Noodle Bowls with Shiitake Mushrooms and Poached Eggs

A bowlful of noodles is a light yet satisfying meal, and these noodle bowls are particularly healthful because they include Brain-Boosting Broth, protein-rich soba noodles, nutrient-dense poached eggs, and green onions, which provide some vitamin C. They're also low in saturated fat. You can put your own unique touches on this dish—for example, try adding some miso to the broth, topping the bowls with some pickled vegetables, or, if you like spicy food, kick up the heat with more chile paste. **MAKES 4 SERVINGS**

1 pound soba noodles

Salt

2 tablespoons white vinegar

4 large eggs, at room temperature

6 cups Brain-Boosting Broth (page 130)

12 fresh shiitake mushrooms, stemmed and sliced ¼ inch thick

2 teaspoons chile paste

1 sheet nori, cut in half on the diagonal

4 green onions, white and green parts, sliced thin

4 teaspoons toasted sesame oil

Fill a large pot two-thirds full with water and bring to a boil over high heat. Add the noodles and cook until al dente. Drain in a colander and divide the noodles among 4 warmed serving bowls.

To poach the eggs, fill a shallow pan with 3 inches of water. Bring the water to a soft boil (180°F) over high heat, then season the water with salt and the white vinegar and turn the heat down to medium-low heat so it is just under a boil. Crack the eggs into individual bowls. Pour each egg into the water slowly, and let poach for 3 minutes, then remove the eggs from the water with a slotted spoon. Let drain.

In the pot you used to cook the noodles, bring the broth to a boil over high heat. Add the mushrooms. Stir in the chile paste.

Ladle the broth with the mushrooms over the four serving bowls with the noodles. Top each bowl with a poached egg, green onions, and nori. Drizzle with 1 teaspoon sesame oil and serve right away.

Sautéed Trout with Wilted Watercress and Oyster Mushroom Salad

Recipes don't get much better than this one for easy preparation and outstanding brain health support. The olive oil provides healthy monounsaturated fat, and the spices and rosemary that season the fish are excellent sources of antioxidants. Watercress also contains antioxidants. But the real star here is the trout, a fish that is high in omega-3 fatty acids for good brain health. Talk to your fishmonger about sourcing best-quality fresh trout, and if whole trout is what's available, ask him or her to fillet the fish for you. **MAKES 4 SERVINGS**

5 tablespoons extra-virgin olive oil

1 teaspoon smoked paprika

1 teaspoon curry powder

1 teaspoon chopped fresh rosemary leaves

4 (6-ounce) skin-on trout fillets

8 ounces oyster mushrooms (1 cup), stemmed and chopped

Salt and freshly ground black pepper

2 bunches watercress, stemmed (about 2 cups)

1 tablespoon minced shallot

1 lemon half

2 tablespoons chopped Herbed Pecans (page 118)

In a small bowl, stir 2 tablespoons of the olive oil with the paprika, curry powder, and rosemary. Lay the trout fillets in a single layer in a shallow baking dish and brush with the oil mixture. Cover and refrigerate for 20 to 60 minutes.

In large sauté pan over medium-high heat, warm 2 tablespoons of the remaining olive oil. Add the mushrooms, season with salt and pepper, and cook, stirring occasionally, until the mushrooms are nicely browned and beginning to crisp, about 2 minutes. Add the watercress and shallots and toss; as soon as the leaves have wilted, transfer the mixture to a large platter. Squeeze the lemon half over the salad.

Return the sauté pan to medium-high heat and warm the remaining 1 tablespoon olive oil. Season the trout fillets with salt and pepper and lay them in the pan and cook for 2 minutes on each side, or until fish flakes easily when tested with a fork. Set the fillets on top of the salad and sprinkle with the pecans. Serve right away.

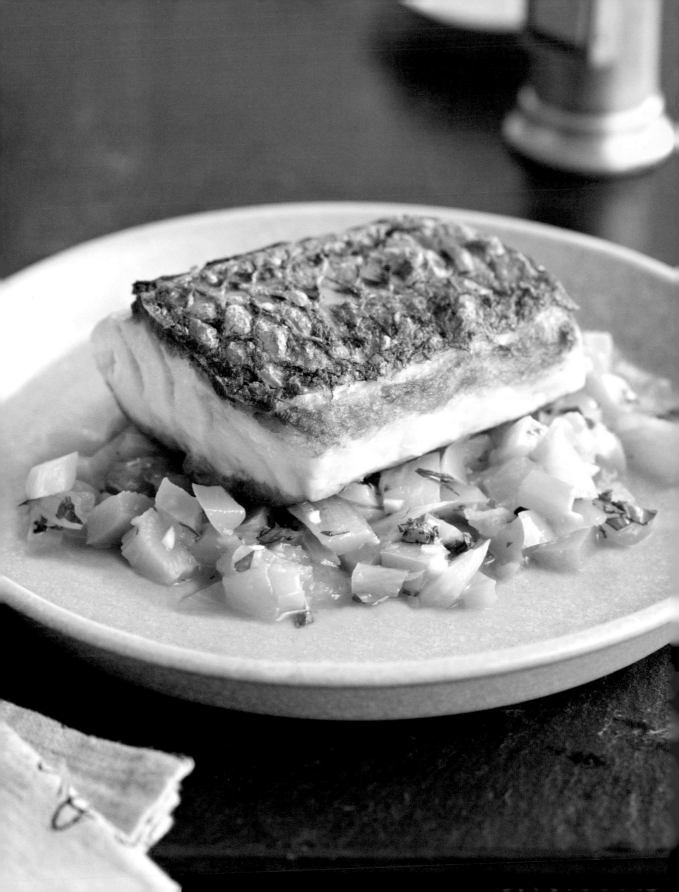

Striped Bass with Golden Tomato and Sweet Pepper Stew

Striped bass provides more than 700 milligrams of omega-3 fatty acids per serving. Put striped bass fillets together with olive oil, which is rich in monounsaturated fat; yellow bell peppers, which are high in polyphenol antioxidants; parsley, an antioxidant herb; and Brain-Boosting Broth, and you get this delicious, colorful, and brain-healthy dish that's also low in saturated fat. If you cannot find striped bass, you can substitute just about any type of skin-on fish fillets, but be sure to make adjustments in the cooking time if the fillets are thinner or thicker than 2 inches. **MAKES 4 SERVINGS**

TOMATO AND SWEET PEPPER STEW

3 tablespoons olive oil

1 tablespoon finely chopped garlic

1 small shallot, finely chopped

1 fennel bulb, diced large

2 yellow bell peppers, seeded and diced large

3 yellow tomatoes, cored and diced large

Pinch of saffron threads

2 tablespoons Pernod or other anise liqueur, such as ouzo or anisette

1 cup white wine

2 cups Brain-Boosting Broth (page 130)

Salt and freshly ground black pepper

FISH

2 tablespoons olive oil

4 (6-ounce) skin-on striped bass fillets

Salt and freshly ground pepper

1 1/2 tablespoons chopped fresh flat-leaf parsley leaves, for garnish

Preheat the oven to 350°F.

To make the stew, in a large saucepan over medium heat, warm the olive oil. Add the garlic, shallot, fennel, and bell peppers and cook, stirring occasionally, until the vegetables soften, about 10 minutes. Add the tomatoes and saffron and continue to cook until the tomatoes soften slightly, about 2 minutes. Pour in the Pernod, bring to a simmer, and cook, stirring, until almost evaporated. Add the white wine, bring to a simmer, and cook until the liquid is reduced by about half, about 5 minutes. Pour in the broth, season with salt and pepper, and simmer uncovered for 15 minutes to bring the flavors together.

While the stew is simmering, cook the fish. In a large ovenproof skillet over medium-high heat, warm the olive oil. Score the fish fillets with a knife and season them with salt and pepper. Add the fish fillets to the skillet skin side down and cook until the skin is golden brown and crisp, about 3 minutes. Slide the skillet into the oven and cook until the fish skin is opaque and flaky, about 5 minutes.

Divide the stew among four plates and place a fish fillet on top. Sprinkle with parsley and serve right away.

Arctic Char with Grilled Red Onion

This-brain healthy dish draws from the Mediterranean region. Adherence to a Mediterranean diet has been shown to be associated with a lower risk of developing Alzheimer's disease. Char—a very tender fish with a mild flavor between salmon and trout—is rich in omega-3 fatty acids, which are important for brain health. Red onion is a good source of polyphenols, and its slight bitterness contrasts nicely with the sweet glaze. MAKES 4 SERVINGS

1 teaspoon fennel seed

1/3 cup orange juice

2 tablespoons rice wine vinegar

1 Tablespoon honey

1 tablespoon brown sugar

2 tablespoons olive oil

1 tablespoon orange zest

4 (6-ounce) arctic char fillets

1 large red onion, sliced into thick rounds

In a small bowl, whisk together the fennel, orange juice, rice vinegar, honey, brown sugar, olive oil, and zest until well combined.

Arrange the char fillets in a shallow pan and pour the glaze over fish. Let the fish marinate for 2 hours.

Build a medium fire on one side of a charcoal grill or heat a gas grill on medium heat. Lay the onion slices on the grill and cook each side until they have nice grill marks and start to soften, 1 to 2 minutes total. Remove the onion from the heat and set aside.

Position an oven rack in the upper third of the oven and preheat the broiler. Place the fish on a rimmed, oiled baking sheet and broil until the fish is lightly browned, or 3 to 4 minutes. Serve with the grilled onion placed alongside the fish.

Grilled Salmon with Molasses-Lime Glaze

Salmon is an excellent source of brain-healthy omega-3 fatty acids. The fish's rich flavor and texture make it an extremely popular and common offering in supermarkets, but when shopping, look for high-quality wild salmon in better grocery stores and fish markets. Since some studies show that eating three fish meals per week is associated with a reduced risk for Alzheimer's disease, it's great to have quick and super-tasty recipes like this one in your repertoire. Steamed jasmine rice is the perfect accompaniment to the grilled glazed fillets. **MAKES 4 SERVINGS**

1 cup dark molasses (not blackstrap)

¼ cup Dijon mustard

Juice of 4 limes

4 teaspoons extra-virgin olive oil, plus more for brushing the salmon

4 teaspoons peeled, minced fresh ginger

4 (6-ounce) skinless wild salmon fillets

Salt and freshly ground black pepper

Build a medium fire on one side of a charcoal grill or heat a gas grill on medium heat.

While the grill heats, in a small bowl, whisk the molasses, mustard, lime juice, olive oil, and ginger until well combined.

Lightly brush both sides of the salmon fillets with olive oil and season with salt and pepper. Lay the fillets over the fire and grill until they get nice grill marks, about 2 minutes. Flip the fillets and continue to grill until the other side has grill marks, about 2 minutes. Flip the fillets and move them to the cooler side of the grill (if using a charcoal grill) or turn down the burners to low (if using a gas grill). Generously brush the surface of each fillet with glaze, cover the grill, and cook until the glaze caramelizes, about 2 minutes. Transfer the fillets to a platter or four serving plates and serve right away.

Salmon and Vegetables Steamed on Banana Leaves

This colorful dish is one of the brain-healthiest dinners that you can put on the table. The salmon is rich in omega-3 fatty acids but low in saturated fat, and the vegetables provide lots of polyphenol antioxidants as well as vitamins. Look for banana leaves for lining the bamboo steamers in Asian markets; if you can't find fresh ones, check in the freezer section for frozen ones. If you happen to own four individual-sized stackable bamboo steamers, you can arrange one serving per steamer so that each person has his or her own bamboo basket at the table (you'll need four banana leaves). Accompany with steamed brown rice, if you like. MAKES 4 SERVINGS

GLAZE

$1/2$ cup soy sauce

$1/2$ cup mirin

$1/2$ cup water

$1/4$ cup rice vinegar

1 tablespoon brown sugar

4 cloves garlic, chopped

2 teaspoons peeled, chopped fresh ginger

2 tablespoons cornstarch

FISH AND VEGETABLES

2 large fresh or thawed frozen banana leaves

5 cups baby spinach (1 pound)

1 small red bell pepper, seeded and cut into matchsticks

1 small yellow bell pepper, seeded and cut into matchsticks

$1/2$ cup shredded napa cabbage

1 large carrot, peeled and cut into matchsticks

8 asparagus spears, sliced in half

8 ($1/2$-inch-thick) slices yellow summer squash

8 ($1/2$-inch-thick) slices zucchini

4 (6-ounce) skinless salmon fillets

4 green onions, white and green parts, sliced thin

Sesame seeds, for garnish

To make the glaze, in small saucepan over medium-high heat, combine the soy sauce, mirin, water, vinegar, brown sugar, garlic, and ginger. Bring to a boil, and then turn down the heat to maintain a gentle simmer. Cook, stirring occasionally, for 5 minutes to blend the flavors.

In a small bowl, stir together the cornstarch and 2 teaspoons water. Stir this cornstarch slurry into the soy sauce mixture and simmer, stirring, until the mixture is clear, glossy, and lightly thickened. Pour the glaze through a fine-mesh sieve set over a bowl.

To steam the fish and vegetables, bring 1 to 2 inches of water to a boil in a large wok. Line the bottom of each of two large stackable bamboo steamers with a banana leaf. Divide the spinach between the steamers, distributing it in an even layer. Divide the red and yellow bell peppers, cabbage, carrot, asparagus, summer squash, and zucchini between the steamers, arranging the vegetables around the perimeter. Set 2 salmon fillets in each steamer, spacing them about $1/2$ inch apart and ensuring they are not covered by the vegetables.

continued

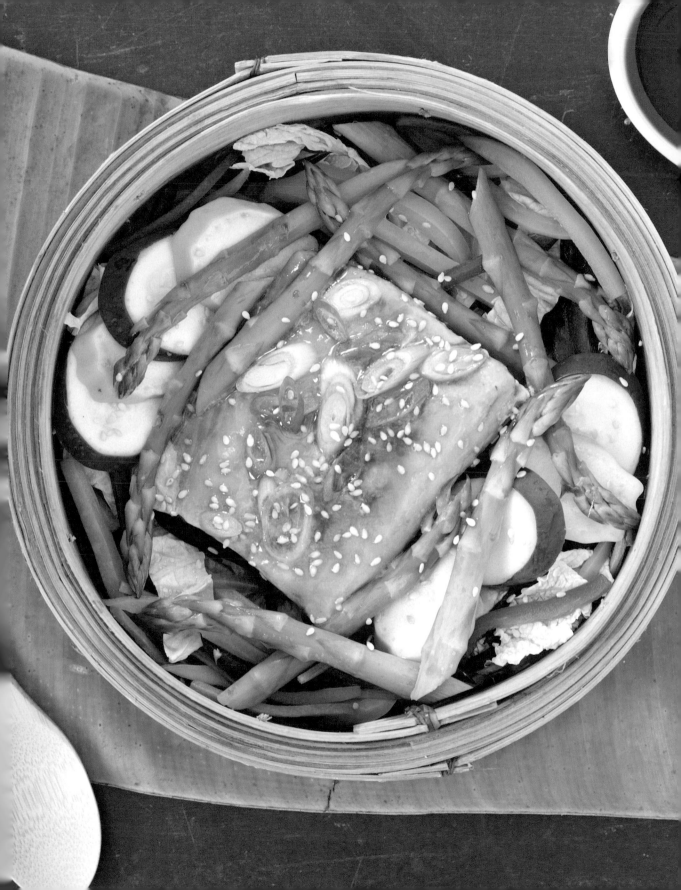

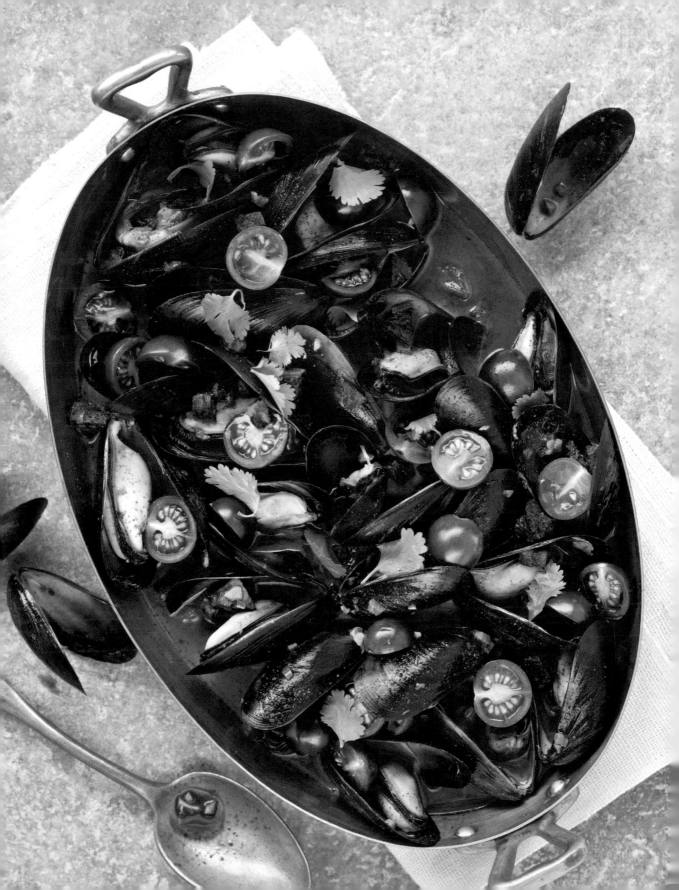

Braised Mussels with Garlic and Chorizo

Mussels are a superb source of vitamin B$_{12}$, an important nutrient for brain health. The sweet, briny flavor of the mollusks pairs perfectly with the spicy, smoky notes of the chorizo. But make sure to use firm, dry-cured Spanish chorizo here, not fresh Mexican-style chorizo. As an added flourish and a dose of healthy monounsaturated fat, you can drizzle each bowl of mussels with good-quality extra-virgin olive oil just before serving. Couscous or quinoa make perfect accompaniments.

MAKES 4 SERVINGS

2 tablespoons extra-virgin olive oil

3 ounces firm Spanish chorizo, chopped

1 tablespoon chopped garlic

1 tablespoon chopped shallot

1 tablespoon smoked paprika

1 teaspoon ground cumin

3 pounds fresh mussels, scrubbed and debearded

$^{1}/_{2}$ cup white wine

$^{1}/_{2}$ cup Brain-Boosting Broth (page 130) or water

1 cup cherry tomatoes (4 ounces), halved

Salt and freshly ground black pepper

1 tablespoon chopped fresh cilantro leaves

1 lime, cut into wedges, for serving

In a Dutch oven over medium-high heat, warm the oil and chorizo. Cook, stirring occasionally, until the chorizo renders some of its fat, about 2 minutes. Stir in the garlic, shallot, paprika, and cumin, followed by the mussels. Pour in the wine, bring to a simmer, and cook, stirring occasionally, until the liquid is reduced by about half, about 3 minutes. Add the broth and continue to cook, covered, until the mussels open, about 3 minutes. Add the tomatoes and season to taste with salt and pepper. Discard any mussels that have not opened.

Spoon the mussels and liquid into four individual bowls, sprinkle with cilantro, and serve right away with lime wedges.

Skewered Pancetta-Wrapped Shrimp with Roasted Bell Pepper Relish

Colossal shrimp may also be known as U-12 or U-10 shrimp, which means that there are fewer than 12 or 10 shrimp per pound. This dish is excellent served with steamed brown rice, and the peppers in the relish add vitamin C. MAKES 4 SERVINGS

RELISH

2 red bell peppers

2 yellow bell peppers

1 medium red onion, diced

1 teaspoon finely chopped garlic

1/2 cup extra-virgin olive oil

2 tablespoons balsamic vinegar

1/4 cup pine nuts, toasted

2 tablespoons chopped fresh flat-leaf parsley leaves

Salt and freshly ground black pepper

SHRIMP

16 thin slices pancetta

16 large fresh basil leaves

16 colossal shrimp, peeled and deveined

Preheat the oven to 375°F. Soak four 8-inch bamboo skewers in water to cover.

Prick the red and yellow bell peppers several times with a fork and set them on a baking sheet. Roast, occasionally turning the peppers with tongs, until the skins are blackened, about 15 minutes. Transfer the peppers to paper bag, close the bag, and let stand for 10 minutes so the steam loosens the skins. Turn down the oven temperature to 350°F.

Peel, seed, and finely chop the peppers. In a medium bowl, combine the peppers, onion, garlic, olive oil, vinegar, pine nuts, and parsley and mix well. Season to taste with salt and pepper. Set the relish aside.

To skewer and cook the shrimp, unfurl the pancetta slices. Working one at a time, wrap a basil leaf around the shrimp, and then wind a slice of pancetta around the basil-wrapped shrimp. Skewer the shrimp, threading them through the tail and head ends, forming a C shape; place 4 shrimp on each skewer.

Warm a large sauté pan over medium-high heat. Lay the skewers in the pan and cook, turning once, until the shrimp are opaque in the center (check by cutting into the widest part of the shrimp) and the pancetta is crisp, about 5 minutes. Transfer the skewers to a rimmed baking sheet and bake until the pancetta is nicely browned, 2 to 3 minutes.

Remove the shrimp from the skewers, arrange the shrimp on a platter, and spoon over the bell pepper relish. Serve right away.

Kimchi-Marinated Steak Salad

This recipe uses flat iron steaks, a cut that is becoming more popular because it offers New York strip steak flavor at a more reasonable price. The steaks are wide and thin, so they're quick to marinate and even quicker to cook. If you can't find flat iron steaks and have asked already asked your butcher, you can use tri-tip instead. Slices of the spicy, warm steak on top of cool, crisp greens (note that spinach is an excellent source of antioxidants) makes for a delicious contrast in flavor and texture.
MAKES 4 SERVINGS

1 cup kimchi, homemade (see page 208) or store-bought

2 (8-ounce) flat iron steaks

1 head red leaf lettuce, roughly chopped

2 cups baby spinach

12 young, slender carrots, peeled and sliced thin

8 ounces (1½ cups) oyster mushrooms, trimmed and chopped

½ cup slivered almonds, toasted

½ cup Soy-Sesame Dressing (page 210)

Salt and freshly ground black pepper

In a blender or food processor, puree the kimchi until smooth. Place the steaks in a shallow baking dish, pour over the kimchi puree, and turn the steaks to coat. Cover and refrigerate for 2 hours.

Build a hot fire in a charcoal grill or heat a gas grill on medium-high heat. When the grill is hot, cook the steaks, turning once, until nicely charred on both sides, 2 to 3 minutes on each side for medium-rare. Let the steaks rest while preparing the salad.

In a large bowl, combine the lettuce, spinach, carrots, mushrooms, and almonds. Drizzle the dressing over, season with salt and pepper, and toss gently. Divide the salad among four serving plates. Cut the steaks against the grain into thin slices and arrange the slices on top of the salads, dividing them evenly. Serve right away.

Grilled Herbed Chicken Breasts with Sesame–Green Onion Rice and Bok Choy

This recipe puts together a main-dish protein, a carbohydrate, and a vegetable to create a brain-healthy meal with Asian flavor accents. The herbs that season the chicken are rich in antioxidants, the brown rice is a delicious way to get a serving of whole grains, and the bok choy is a great source of a number of different vitamins, especially vitamins A and C. Beau recommends using boneless chicken breast halves with the skin still attached so that the meat stays extra flavorful and juicy, even after cooking on a hot grill. If the only skin-on chicken breasts you can find are sold with the bone, you can debone them yourself or ask the butcher to do it for you.

MAKES 4 SERVINGS

CHICKEN

1 tablespoon chopped fresh thyme leaves

1 tablespoon chopped fresh rosemary leaves

2 tablespoons extra-virgin olive oil

1 teaspoon salt

1 teaspoon freshly ground black pepper

4 (6-ounce) boneless, skin-on chicken breasts, trimmed

RICE

1 1/2 cups brown rice

3 cups water

2 tablespoons extra-virgin olive oil

1/2 medium red onion, diced small

8 green onions, white and green parts, chopped

2 tablespoons toasted sesame oil

Splash of rice vinegar

Salt and freshly ground black pepper

To marinate the chicken, in a medium bowl or baking dish, combine the thyme, rosemary, olive oil, salt, and pepper. Add the chicken breasts and turn to coat. Cover and refrigerate for at least 1 hour or up to 6 hours.

To prepare the rice, rinse the rice in a fine-mesh sieve under running water until the water runs clear. Put the rice in a medium saucepan and add the water. Bring to a boil over medium-high heat, cover, and turn down the heat to maintain a gentle simmer. Cook until the rice is tender and plump, about 25 minutes. Let rest, covered, for 10 minutes.

While the rice is cooking, warm the olive oil in a small skillet over medium heat. Add the red onion and cook, stirring occasionally, until softened, about 5 minutes. Add the onion to a medium bowl.

Transfer the cooked rice to the bowl with the sautéed red onion and add the green onions, sesame oil, and rice vinegar. Stir to combine and season to taste with salt and pepper. Cover to keep warm.

BOK CHOY

4 heads baby bok choy

2 tablespoons extra-virgin
   olive oil

2 tablespoons peeled,
   chopped
   fresh ginger

1 tablespoon chopped garlic

2 green onions, sliced on
   the diagonal, for garnish

To grill the chicken, build a medium-hot fire in a charcoal grill or heat a gas grill on medium-high heat. When the grill is hot, cook the chicken breasts, turning once, until nicely browned on both sides and the center of the thickest part registers 160°F on an instant-read thermometer, 6 to 8 minutes. Let rest while preparing the bok choy.

To prepare the bok choy, in a large skillet over medium heat, warm the olive oil. Add the ginger and garlic and cook, stirring, until fragrant, about 30 seconds. Add the bok choy and cook, tossing occasionally, until heated through and the flavors have blended, 2 to 3 minutes. Add $1/4$ cup water (stand back when adding the water to the skillet) to finish cooking and steaming the bok choy until it is soft.

To serve, divide the rice, bok choy, and chicken among four dinner plates. Garnish with the green onions and serve right away.

Roasted Chicken Breasts with Spicy Beluga Lentils

With a combination of boneless, skinless chicken breasts and lentils, this dish packs in lots of lean, healthy protein with very minimal amounts of saturated fat. The onion, herbs, and spices bring big, bold flavor to the lentils, and, along with the Brain-Boosting Broth, are great sources of brain-healthy antioxidants. Beluga lentils are so named because they're small, black, and resemble caviar. Look for them in well-stocked grocery stores; if you can't find them, French green lentils are a good substitute, but they will take slightly longer to cook, or any other lentils can work, in a pinch. **MAKES 4 SERVINGS**

3 tablespoons extra-virgin olive oil, plus more to rub chicken

1 medium yellow onion, chopped

4 cloves garlic, minced

4 jalapeño chiles, seeded and chopped

2 teaspoons ground cumin

2 teaspoons dried oregano

1 teaspoon red pepper flakes

2 tablespoons paprika

2 cups beluga lentils

6 cups Brain-Boosting Broth (page 130)

Salt and freshly ground black pepper

4 (6-ounce) boneless, skinless chicken breasts, trimmed

2 tablespoons chopped fresh cilantro leaves

Preheat the oven to 350°F.

In a large saucepan over medium-high heat, warm the olive oil. Add the onion, garlic, jalapeños, cumin, oregano, and red pepper flakes and cook, stirring occasionally, until they soften, about 3 minutes. Add the paprika, lentils, and broth; increase the heat to high; and bring to a boil. Cover, turn down the heat to maintain a simmer, and cook until the lentils are tender, 15 to 20 minutes. Season to taste with salt and pepper.

While the lentils are cooking, rub the chicken breasts with olive oil and season with salt and pepper. Place the breasts in a single layer on a small rimmed baking sheet or in a shallow baking dish and roast until the center of the thickest part registers 160°F on an instant-read thermometer, 10 to 12 minutes. Let rest for 5 minutes.

Spoon the lentils onto four serving plates or into shallow bowls. Cut the chicken crosswise into slices and lay the slices on top of the lentils. Sprinkle with cilantro and serve right away.

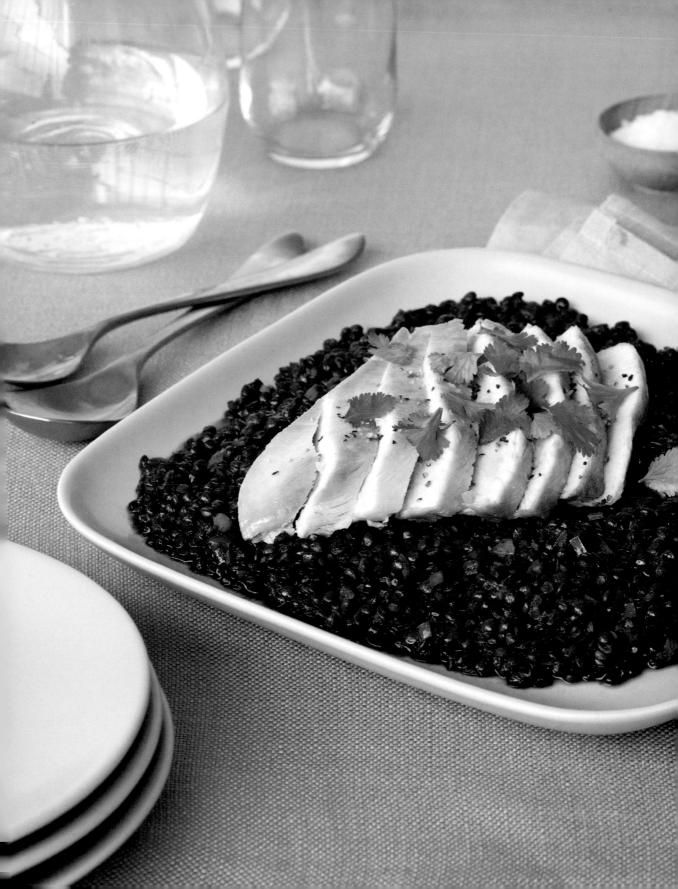

Braised Short Ribs with Root Vegetables and Kale

This recipe uses Brain-Boosting Broth as part of the cooking liquid. During braising, the already-antioxidant-rich broth is fortified with additional vegetables and herbs as well as with red wine (which contains resveratrol), and then in the final stage of cooking, four different kinds of root vegetables and nutrient-dense kale are added. All this adds up to one very brain-healthy meal. But the recipe does require time investment: short ribs need long, slow simmering to make them tender, so plan ahead if you make this dish, and don't rush the cooking. MAKES 4 SERVINGS

SHORT RIBS

2 tablespoons extra-virgin olive oil

2 pounds boneless beef short ribs, trimmed and cut into 3-inch cubes

Salt and freshly ground black pepper

3 medium carrots, peeled and chopped

2 celery stalks, chopped

2 medium yellow onions, chopped

1/2 cup whole peeled garlic cloves

10 sprigs thyme

1 tablespoon black peppercorns

1 bay leaf

1 cup red wine

1 gallon Brain-Boosting Broth (page 130)

Preheat the oven to 300°F.

To make the short ribs, in a large, heavy-bottomed Dutch oven over high heat, warm the oil. Season the ribs with salt and pepper, add the short ribs to the Dutch oven, and sear on all sides until well browned, about 5 minutes. Transfer the ribs to a plate. Add the carrots, celery, and onions and cook, stirring occasionally, until browned, 3 to 5 minutes. Add the garlic, thyme, peppercorns, and bay leaf and cook for 1 minute. Return the ribs to the Dutch oven, pour in the wine, and scrape up any browned bits on the bottom of the pot. Bring the wine to a simmer and cook until reduced to about 1/2 cup. Pour in the broth, increase the heat to high, and bring to a boil. Cover, place the Dutch oven in the oven, and cook until the short ribs are fork-tender, 2 1/2 to 3 hours.

To cook the vegetables and finish the dish, transfer the ribs to a plate. Strain the braising liquid through a fine-mesh sieve into a second Dutch oven or soup pot. Allow the stew to rest for 1 hour in the

VEGETABLES

2 sweet potatoes (about 8 ounces each), peeled and cut into 1-inch chunks

1 medium carrot, cut into $\frac{1}{2}$-inch pieces

1 medium yellow onion, chopped

1 turnip (about 8 ounces), peeled and chopped

2 tablespoons peeled, chopped fresh ginger

1 tablespoon chopped garlic

2 cups shredded kale leaves

Salt and freshly ground black pepper

refrigerator so that the fat rises to the surface, and then skim off the fat with a spoon. Return the stew to the stove, bring to a simmer over medium-high heat, and add the sweet potatoes, carrot, onion, turnip, ginger, and garlic. Cover and cook until a fork inserted into a piece of carrot or turnip meets no resistance, about 10 minutes. Stir in the kale and simmer until the leaves are tender, about 5 minutes. Nestle the short ribs in the pot, cover, and cook just until the meat is heated through, about 5 minutes. Season to taste with salt and pepper.

Transfer the meat, vegetables, and sauce to four warmed serving bowls and serve right away.

Lamb Stew with Fragrant Spices

This robustly flavored stew draws on the cooking of the Indian subcontinent region where the incidence of Alzheimer's disease is among the lowest in the world. The brain-health benefits of this dish come from the antioxidant-rich spices and the Brain-Boosting Broth. Braises like this one take some time to cook but are well worth the wait—you'll be rewarded with moist, tender meat in a rich sauce. Try serving this stew with some crusty whole-grain bread to soak up the liquid. MAKES 4 SERVINGS

¼ cup extra-virgin olive oil

2 teaspoons cumin seed

3 tablespoons peeled, finely chopped fresh ginger

2 large white onions, thinly sliced

2 pounds boneless lamb shoulder, trimmed and cut into 1½-inch chunks

1 tablespoon paprika

2 teaspoons ground coriander

1½ teaspoons ground turmeric

1 teaspoon curry powder

1 teaspoon cayenne pepper

Pinch of salt

½ cup low-fat or nonfat plain yogurt

2 cups Brain Boosting Broth (page 130)

½ cup sliced roasted almonds

2 tablespoons chopped fresh cilantro leaves

In a large, heavy-bottomed Dutch oven over medium-high heat, warm the olive oil. Add the cumin seed and ginger and stir rapidly until fragrant. Add the onions and cook, stirring occasionally, until the onions have softened, 10 to 15 minutes. Add the lamb and cook, stirring occasionally, until browned evenly and any moisture in the Dutch oven has evaporated, 3 to 4 minutes. Stir in the paprika, coriander, turmeric, curry powder, cayenne, and salt and cook until the spices are fragrant, about 2 minutes. Remove from the heat and let the mixture cool until just warm to the touch, about 10 minutes, so that the yogurt does not curdled when added.

Add the yogurt to the Dutch oven and stir rapidly to prevent it from curdling. Return the Dutch oven to medium heat and pour in the broth. Increase the heat to medium-high, and bring the stew to maintain a simmer. Cover and cook, stirring occasionally, until the lamb is fork-tender, 25 to 30 minutes.

Ladle the stew into four serving bowls, garnish with almonds and cilantro, and serve right away.

CHAPTER 14

Vegetables, Grains, and Legumes

Roasted Onions with Rosemary and Tamarind Vinegar

In this brain-healthy recipe, the turmeric in the curry powder delivers robust anti-inflammatory and antioxidant qualities. The dish also contains olive oil, a good source of monounsaturated fat, and rosemary, a potent antioxidant herb. Beau recommends using sweet onions, such as Vidalia, Maui, and Walla Walla, because their mild flavor and high sugar content make an especially tasty dish. Sweet onions are usually available in the spring and summer. If you can't find tamarind vinegar (look online or in specialty grocery stores), you can use any other type of vinegar. The roasted onions are a delicious accompaniment to meats and poultry, but they're also great on top of dressed greens as part of a salad. MAKES 6 SERVINGS

6 medium sweet onions, peeled and quartered lengthwise (keep the root end intact)

3 tablespoons extra-virgin olive oil

2½ tablespoons tamarind vinegar, other vinegar, or freshly squeezed lemon juice

1½ tablespoons chopped fresh rosemary leaves

1 tablespoon curry powder

1 tablespoon grated orange zest

¼ cup water

Salt and freshly ground black pepper

Preheat the oven to 375°F.

In a shallow baking dish or roasting pan, toss the onions, olive oil, vinegar, rosemary, curry powder, and orange zest. Pour the water into the dish, cover with aluminum foil, and roast for 30 minutes.

Remove the foil and continue to roast until the onion are fully tender and nicely browned, about 5 minutes. Serve warm.

Super-Simple Ratatouille

Ratatouille is a dish that's very typical of the brain-healthy Mediterranean diet. The wide variety of dark-colored vegetables that goes into this recipe provides vitamins C and E as well as beta-carotene and polyphenol antioxidants, and the olive oil supplies monounsaturated fat. In this version, Beau's quick and easy take on traditional ratatouille, the vegetables are cooked only briefly, so they retain their freshness and bright flavor. You can serve ratatouille as a side dish to proteins like grilled chicken, use it as a filling for omelets (see the recipe on page 112), or with some polenta as a vegetarian main dish. MAKES ABOUT 3 CUPS, SERVING 4

1 globe eggplant (about 12 ounces), diced into ¼-inch cubes

1 zucchini, diced into ¼-inch cubes

1 yellow summer squash, diced into ¼-inch cubes

1 red bell pepper, seeded and diced into ¼-inch cubes

1 yellow bell pepper, seeded and diced into ¼-inch cubes

1 large red onion, diced into ¼-inch cubes

2 tablespoons extra-virgin olive oil

2 tablespoons finely chopped garlic

2 tablespoons shredded fresh basil leaves

Salt and freshly ground black pepper

2 ripe tomatoes (about 8 ounces total), cored and diced medium

In a large bowl, combine the eggplant, zucchini, summer squash, red and yellow pepper bell peppers, and onion. Drizzle with the olive oil and toss to coat.

Heat a large sauté pan, preferably cast iron, over high heat. Add the vegetable mixture and cook, stirring occasionally, until lightly softened, about 2 minutes. Stir in the garlic and basil and season to taste with salt and pepper. Fold in the tomatoes and remove from the heat. Serve warm or at room temperature.

Roasted Corn on the Cob in Spicy Red Pepper Puree

This is a fun, super-delicious, family-friendly recipe to make in the summer, when corn is in season. The roasted bell peppers and sun-dried tomatoes bolster the corn's natural sweetness while the chipotle chile adds some snappy smoke and spice, so although the dish is low in saturated fat, it's big on flavor. The red bell peppers, fresh corn, and sun-dried tomatoes provide vitamin C, polyphenol antioxidants, and vitamin B$_6$ for good brain health. **MAKES 6 SERVINGS**

2 medium red bell peppers

2 oil-packed sun-dried tomatoes, patted dry and coarsely chopped

1 chipotle chile in adobo sauce

6 green onions, chopped

1 shallot, coarsely chopped

1 clove garlic, coarsely chopped

1 tablespoon light brown sugar

6 ears fresh corn, husks pulled back but attached, silk removed

Salt and freshly ground black pepper

Roast the red bell peppers in the oven at 375°F on a baking sheet, on the grill, or held with tongs over a flame on a gas oven. Char the skin, rotating it for even charring, for 5 to 8 minutes. Once the skin starts cracking, place the pepper in a small bowl and cover the bowl with plastic wrap for 5 minutes. The skin will steep and separate from the peppers so that you can peel it off easily. Once the peppers are cool, peel and seed them, then coarsely chop.

Add the peppers to a blender or food processor along with the sun-dried tomatoes, chipotle chile, green onions, shallot, garlic, and brown sugar and puree until smooth.

Place the ears of corn in a large pot of water and let soak for 30 minutes before roasting.

Build a medium-hot fire in a charcoal grill, heat a gas grill on medium-high heat, or preheat the oven to 500°F.

Using a small metal spoon or your hands, spread red-pepper puree all over the ears of corn, dividing it evenly, and pulling the husk back to spread the puree directly onto the kernels, then replacing the husk. Season with salt and pepper.

Roast the corn on the grill, covered, or in the oven directly on the oven rack (you might want to place a baking sheet on the rack underneath the ears to catch any puree that drips down) for 20 minutes, rotating the corn halfway through to ensure even roasting, or until the kernels are completely tender.

Unwrap each ear, remove and discard the husk (or serve in the husk, if you like), and serve. Season again with salt and pepper, to taste.

Sautéed Mushrooms with Spinach and Black Vinegar

This dish is full of rich, earthy, meaty flavors from the mushrooms and aromatics, but it's low in saturated fat, contains polyphenol antioxidants from the spinach, and has monounsaturated fat from the olive oil, so it's good for brain health. Beau's favorite combination of mushrooms to use is oyster, shiitake, and maitake mushrooms, but you can use any types you prefer. Black vinegar has a rich but mild taste and is usually made from rice or millet. **MAKES 6 SERVINGS**

2 tablespoons olive oil

1 pound mixed mushrooms, preferably oyster, shiitake, and maitake mushrooms, trimmed and quartered

5 medium shallots, finely chopped

1 tablespoon finely chopped garlic

1 tablespoon peeled, chopped fresh ginger

Salt and freshly ground black pepper

2 tablespoons Chinese black vinegar or sherry vinegar

1 cup spinach

In a large, heavy-bottomed skillet over high heat, warm the olive oil. Add the mushrooms and cook, stirring frequently, until charred and crispy brown on the outside, about 2 minutes. Add the shallots, garlic, and ginger and continue to cook until the mushrooms have browned, about 2 minutes longer. Season with salt and pepper to taste before pouring in the black vinegar, and cook, scraping up any browned bits, until the moisture has evaporated. Fold in the spinach and season with salt and pepper to taste. Transfer to a bowl and serve.

Broiled Japanese Eggplant with Miso

Eggplant is an excellent source of polyphenol antioxidants; the antioxidants reside mostly in the skin. In this recipe, be sure to use small, dark-skinned Japanese eggplants; large, bulbous globe eggplants are seedy and won't cook through properly. If you can find black or fermented garlic, use 2 tablespoons mashed to a paste in place of the regular garlic. This side dish is excellent alongside steak or lamb dishes.

MAKES 4 SERVINGS

4 Japanese eggplants, cut lengthwise in half
Salt
2 tablespoons minced garlic
1/4 cup water
2 tablespoons white miso
3 tablespoons soy sauce
1 tablespoon mirin
1 teaspoon rice vinegar
1 teaspoon Asian chile paste
1 teaspoon toasted sesame oil
Pinch of ground Szechuan pepper
Cilantro sprigs, for garnish (optional)

Score the eggplant flesh with a knife or pierce several times with a fork. Place the eggplant halves cut side up in a single layer in a shallow baking dish and sprinkle each half lightly with salt. Let stand at room temperature for 45 minutes.

In a small bowl, stir the garlic, water, miso, soy sauce, mirin, vinegar, chile paste, sesame oil, and Szechuan pepper until well combined.

Using paper towels, wipe the salt off the eggplant and pat dry. Spread the miso mixture over the cut side of the eggplant halves, cover, and refrigerate for 1 1/2 hours.

Position an oven rack 8 to 10 inches from the broiler and preheat the broiler. Uncover the baking dish and broil until the eggplant is tender and creamy, 8 to 10 minutes.

Using a spatula, transfer the eggplant halves to a platter and serve.

Sautéed Butternut Squash with Charred Shishito Peppers

Shishito peppers are small, green Japanese chiles. They can be spicy hot, or not: it's been said that one out of every ten shishito peppers packs a punch. Beau likes to char them to bring out their flavor and add a touch of smokiness. (If you can't find shishitos, substitute Anaheim or poblano chiles.) Here, he adds charred shishitos to sautéed butternut squash. The combination of sweetness and spiciness is highly addictive. This dish not only tastes good, it's good for you and your brain. It's very low in saturated fat, is rich in vitamin A from the butternut squash, and contains a dose of antioxidants from the thyme. MAKES 4 TO 6 SERVINGS

8 ounces shishito peppers, stemmed and sliced into 1/4-inch rings (2 cups)

5 tablespoons extra-virgin olive oil

2 large butternut squash (about 24 ounces each), peeled, seeded, and diced (about 3 cups)

1 medium shallot, minced

2 cloves garlic, minced

1 teaspoon ground coriander

1/2 teaspoon ground cumin

1 tablespoon chopped fresh thyme leaves

Salt and freshly ground black pepper

Position an oven rack 8 to 10 inches from the broiler and preheat the broiler. Distribute the shishito peppers in an even layer on a rimmed baking sheet and broil until the peppers are nicely charred, about 3 minutes. Stir the peppers once, about halfway through the broiling. Set the peppers aside.

In a medium sauté pan over medium-high heat, warm the olive oil and add the diced squash, stirring frequently until the squash begins to soften, about 5 minutes. Add the shishito peppers and stir frequently for 6 to 8 minutes longer until they begin to brown and blister. Add the shallot and garlic and cook, stirring frequently, until golden brown, about 1 minute. Add the coriander, cumin, and thyme and toss to combine. Cook, stirring occasionally, until the mixture is heated through, 3 to 4 minutes. Season with salt and pepper to taste. Serve right away.

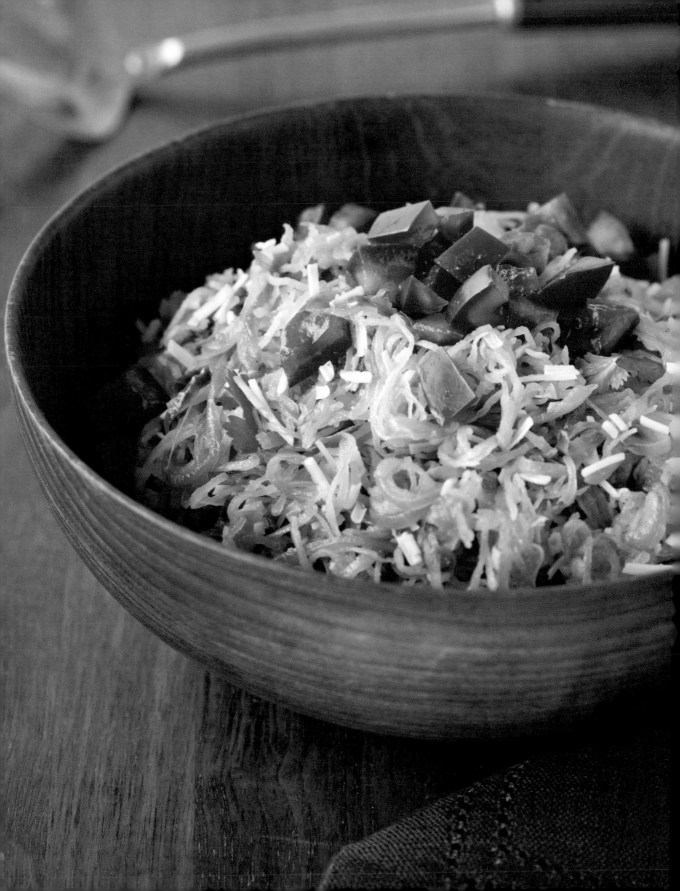

Spaghetti Squash with Caramelized Onion and Tomato

Spaghetti squash is an often-overlooked vegetable. But it's a very powerful ingredient from a brain-health perspective: it's low in saturated fat, very low in cholesterol, and a good source of niacin, vitamin B6, and pantothenic acid—plus spaghetti squash is a very good source of vitamin C. In this recipe, strands of baked spaghetti squash are the backdrop for sweet caramelized onions that contrast against salty, savory Parmesan cheese. This dish will appeal to adults and kids alike, and it's a great way to get pasta lovers to eat more vegetables. **MAKES 4 SERVINGS**

Olive oil

1/2 spaghetti squash (about 2 pounds), seeded

1 tablespoon unsalted butter

1 medium yellow onion, thinly sliced

Curry Salt (page 206)

1/2 cup grated Parmigiano-Reggiano cheese

1/3 cup chopped fresh chives

1 ripe tomato, cored, seeded, and diced

Fresh cilantro leaves, for garnish

Preheat the oven to 350°F.

Drizzle a rimmed baking sheet and the flesh of the squash with a little olive oil. Set the squash half cut side down on the baking sheet. Sprinkle 2 tablespoons of water over the squash and bake, uncovered, until a fork inserted into the thickest part of the flesh meets no resistance, 30 to 45 minutes. Let cool to room temperature.

In a large nonstick skillet over medium heat, melt the butter. Add the onion and cook, stirring occasionally, until lightly caramelized, about 5 minutes. Set aside.

Using a fork, scrape the squash from the skin into a medium bowl; the flesh will separate into spaghetti-like strands (you should have about 2 1/2 cups). Return the skillet with the onion to medium heat and add the squash. Cook, tossing gently, just until heated through, 1 to 2 minutes. Season to taste with Curry Salt; go easy because the cheese will add salt, too. Toss in the cheese and chives and transfer to a serving bowl. Sprinkle with the tomatoes and cilantro and serve right away.

Spicy Butternut Squash Puree with Chinese Five-Spice and Honey

Roasted and pureed butternut squash is delicious on its own, but this recipe incorporates a few ingredients to really kick up the flavor. Honey adds a direct, up-front sweetness, and chipotle chiles in adobo and Chinese five-spice powder bring dimensions in smoke and spice that linger on the palate. Butternut squash looks good, tastes great, and with lots of vitamin C and low amounts of saturated fat, it's healthy for your brain, too. MAKES 6 SERVINGS

2 large butternut squash (about 24 ounces each), cut lengthwise in half and seeded

1 tablespoon extra-virgin olive oil

1 can chipotle chiles in adobo

1 tablespoon Chinese five-spice powder

1 tablespoon honey

Salt and freshly ground black pepper

Preheat the oven to 350°F. Line a rimmed baking sheet with parchment paper.

Rub the squash halves all over with the olive oil and set them cut side down on the prepared baking sheet. Bake until a fork inserted into the thickest part of the flesh meets no resistance, 30 to 35 minutes. Let cool slightly.

Puree the chipotle chiles in adobo in a blender or food processor, both the liquid and peppers, to create a paste. Reserve 1 teaspoon, plus more to taste, and refrigerate the remaining paste. Extra paste will keep for 2 weeks in an airtight container in the refrigerator.

Turn the squash halves cut side up. Using a spoon, scoop the flesh from the skin and add it to a medium bowl. Add the adobo paste, five-spice powder, honey, and salt and pepper to taste, and mash with a fork until well combined. Serve right away.

Balsamic Roasted Vegetables

This recipe is a beautiful medley of roasted vegetables. You'll find lots of different flavor profiles, such as bitterness from the rutabaga, earthiness from the parsnips, and sweetness from the onions, as well as a variety of textures, like hearty and firm carrots, yielding zucchini, and meaty mushrooms. The balsamic vinegar adds a little acidity and helps the vegetables develop rich, flavorful caramelization.

Parsnips are a particularly brain-healthy root vegetable: it's an excellent source of vitamin C and folic acid. It is also a good source of riboflavin, niacin, and vitamins B_6 and E. MAKES 6 TO 8 SERVINGS

1 tablespoon extra-virgin olive oil

1 tablespoon balsamic vinegar

2 carrots, peeled and cut on the diagonal into 1/2-inch pieces

2 parsnips, peeled and cut on the diagonal into 1/2-inch pieces

1/2 medium rutabaga (about 4 ounces), peeled and cut into 1/4-inch chunks

6 pearl onions, peeled, or 1 medium red onion, cut into 8 wedges

Salt and freshly ground black pepper

2 Japanese eggplants, cut lengthwise in half, and then crosswise in half

1 medium zucchini, cut lengthwise in half, and then crosswise in thirds

1 medium yellow summer squash, cut lengthwise in half, and then crosswise in thirds

1 large tomato, cored, seeded, and diced large

3 portobello mushrooms, stems removed, caps cut in half

1 teaspoon fresh thyme leaves

Place a large roasting pan in the oven and preheat the oven to 500°F.

In a small bowl, combine the olive oil and vinegar. In a large bowl, toss the carrots, parsnips, rutabaga, and onions. Whisk the olive oil–vinegar mixture to recombine, drizzle 1 tablespoon over the vegetables, and sprinkle with salt and pepper. Toss well to coat. Transfer the vegetables to the hot roasting pan, distributing them in an even layer. Roast, uncovered, for 8 to 10 minutes, or until the vegetables have softened and can be pierced with a fork. Stir the vegetables occasionally while roasting.

In the now-empty bowl, toss the eggplants, zucchini, summer squash, tomato, and mushrooms. Drizzle with the remaining olive oil–vinegar mixture, sprinkle with salt and pepper, and toss well to coat. Add this vegetable mixture to the roasting pan and roast for about 20 minutes, or until all the vegetables are tender and caramelized, stirring occasionally.

Stir the thyme into the roasted vegetables. Transfer to a large serving bowl and serve right away.

Roasted Carrots

Carrots are supercharged with brain-healthy vitamin A, and their natural sweetness means they taste great, too. If you can, shop for carrots at your farmers' market; there, you'll likely find an array of varieties ranging in color from white to purple. Roasting concentrates vegetables' flavor, so this recipe is a wonderful way to showcase farm-fresh, locally grown carrots. **MAKES 6 SERVINGS**

10 carrots, peeled and cut on the diagonal into 1/2-inch pieces

1 tablespoon extra-virgin olive oil

Salt and freshly ground black pepper

1 tablespoon unsalted butter

1 1/2 teaspoons finely chopped shallot

1 clove garlic, finely chopped

1 1/2 teaspoons chopped fresh flat-leaf parsley leaves

Place a small roasting pan in the oven and preheat the oven to 400°F.

Add the carrots to a bowl, drizzle with the olive oil, and sprinkle with salt and pepper. Toss well to coat. Transfer the carrots onto the hot roasting pan, distributing them in an even layer. Roast, uncovered, stirring occasionally for 10 minutes, or until lightly softened. Let cool until ready to serve.

When ready to serve, in a large skillet over medium heat, melt the butter. Add the shallot, garlic, parsley, and carrots and cook, stirring frequently, until the carrots are fully tender, 3 to 4 minutes. Serve right away.

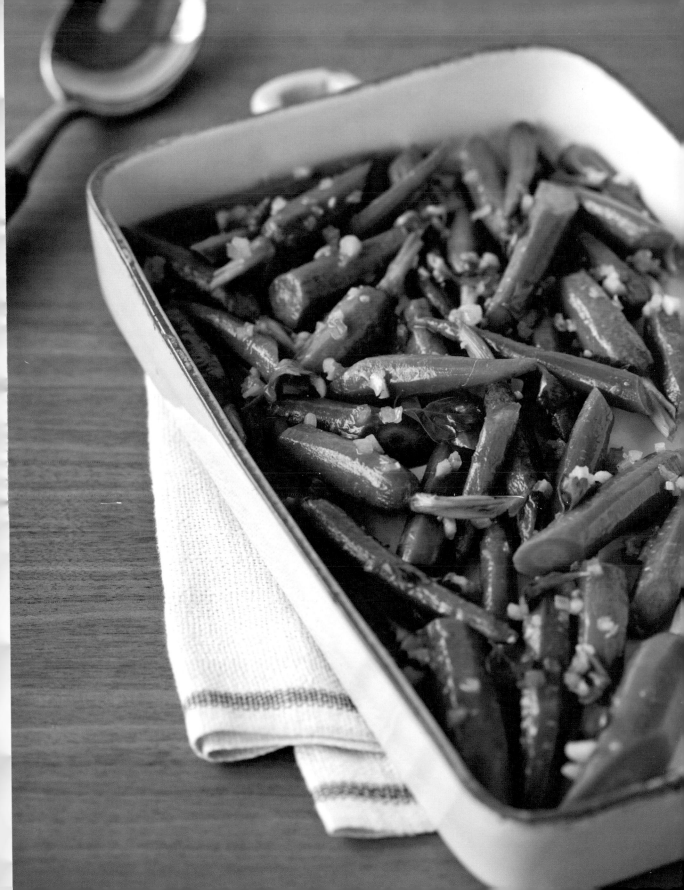

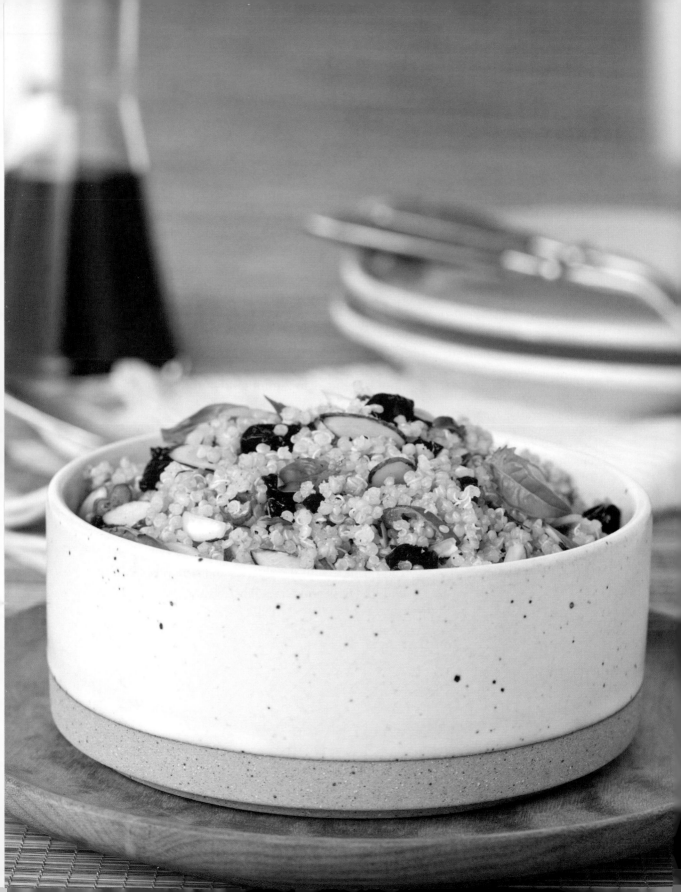

Curried Quinoa with Green Onions and Basil

Quinoa is a grainlike seed that's an excellent source of complete protein. Make sure to simmer your quinoa until it's nice and tender—the texture in this dish should come from the toasted almonds, not al dente quinoa. With monounsaturated fat from the olive oil, antioxidants from the basil and turmeric (in the curry powder), polyphenol antioxidants from the dried cherries, vitamin E from the almonds, and the nutrients of Brain-Boosting Broth, it's hard to imagine a side dish that's better for you and your brain than this one (which also happens to be low in saturated fat).

MAKES 4 SERVINGS

1½ cups Brain-Boosting Broth (page 130)

¾ cup quinoa, rinsed

1 teaspoon curry powder

1 teaspoon minced fresh ginger

5 to 7 green onions, white and green parts, chopped

¼ cup chopped fresh basil leaves

¼ cup slivered almonds, toasted

¼ cup dried cherries, chopped

Pinch of salt

Pinch of freshly ground black pepper

Juice of 1 lemon

2 tablespoons extra-virgin olive oil

In a medium saucepan over high heat, bring the broth to a boil. Add the quinoa, curry powder, and ginger. Turn down the heat to medium-low, cover, and simmer until the quinoa is tender, about 20 minutes.

Transfer the quinoa to a rimmed baking sheet, distribute in an even layer, and let cool to room temperature. When cooled, put the quinoa into a medium bowl and add the green onions, basil, almonds, and cherries. Sprinkle with the salt and pepper and toss to combine. Drizzle with the lemon juice and olive oil and toss again. Serve at room temperature or lightly chilled.

Wild Rice with Root Vegetables

In the Mediterranean diet, whole grains are preferred alternatives to simple carbo-hydrates. This recipe combines a whole grain—naturally nutty-tasting wild rice—with onion, a source of polyphenol antioxidants; carrots that are full of vitamin A; parsley and sage, antioxidant herbs; and the nutrient-rich Brain-Boosting Broth for a very brain-healthy side dish. Dried figs give the rice a sweet-savory quality that's delicious with just about any type of protein, from fish to lamb. MAKES 6 SERVINGS

3 tablespoons extra-virgin olive oil

1 medium celery root (about 6 ounces), peeled and diced small

2 small carrots, peeled and diced small

1 medium white onion, diced small

1½ cups wild rice

5 cups Brain-Boosting Broth (page 130)

½ teaspoon salt

½ teaspoon freshly ground black pepper

¼ cup chopped dried figs

2 tablespoons chopped fresh flat-leaf parsley leaves

1 teaspoon chopped fresh sage leaves

¼ cup pine nuts, toasted

In a large saucepan over medium heat, warm the olive oil. Add the celery root, carrots, and onion and cook, stirring occasionally, until the vegetables soften, about 3 minutes. Add the wild rice and continue to cook, stirring occasionally, for about 2 minutes, or until well coated and incorporated. Pour in the broth and add the salt and pepper. Increase the heat to medium-high, bring the mixture to a boil, and then turn down the heat to maintain a simmer. Cover and cook until the rice is tender, about 45 minutes.

Add the figs, parsley, sage, and pine nuts and toss to combine and fluff the grains. Serve right away.

Israeli Couscous with Mango, Almonds, and Baby Spinach

This recipe may call for Israeli couscous, but the flavors are inspired by Indian cuisine. The curry powder contains turmeric, a spice with potent antioxidant and anti-inflammatory properties that has been credited in contributing to the lower incidence of Alzheimer's disease in India. The spinach, onion, and raisins all add polyphenol antioxidants to the dish, and the mango supplies vitamin C. If you're trying to incorporate more whole grains into your diet, you can replace the couscous (which is a type of pasta) with 2 cups of cooked brown rice, millet, or quinoa.

MAKES 4 TO 6 SERVINGS

2¹/₂ cups water

2 cups Israeli couscous

1 cup peeled, chopped ripe mango

1 medium red onion, chopped

¹/₄ cup fresh cilantro leaves

2 tablespoons champagne vinegar

2 tablespoons freshly squeezed orange juice

1¹/₂ teaspoons Dijon mustard

1 tablespoon curry powder

Pinch of ground coriander

¹/₂ cup low-fat or nonfat plain yogurt

¹/₄ cup golden raisins

¹/₄ cup slivered almonds, toasted

1 cup baby spinach

Salt and freshly ground black pepper

In a medium pot over high heat, bring the water to a boil. Add the couscous and turn down the heat to maintain a simmer. Cover and cook, stirring occasionally, for 8 to 10 minutes. Let the couscous cool for about 10 minutes.

In a food processor or blender, pulse the mango, onion, cilantro, vinegar, orange juice, mustard, curry powder, and coriander until it has the consistency of a vinaigrette and is evenly incorporated. Transfer the mixture to a medium bowl and stir in the yogurt. Add the raisins, almonds, spinach, and couscous. Stir well to combine, season to taste with salt and pepper, and serve.

Red Lentils and Kale with Miso

This dish draws on both Mediterranean and Asian influences and uses the very different flavors of sage, miso, and nori in complementary ways. It's a brain-healthy recipe: legumes such as lentils are a key component of the Mediterranean diet, both kale and onions are good sources of polyphenol antioxidants, and sweet potato supplies a dose of beta-carotene. MAKES 4 TO 6 SERVINGS

1 cup dried red lentils, rinsed

4 cups Brain-Boosting Broth (page 130)

3 cloves garlic, chopped

1 sweet potato, peeled and chopped

2 celery stalks, chopped

1 yellow onion, chopped

2 cups Roma tomatoes, chopped

1 tablespoon white miso

1 bunch kale, stemmed and chopped

Salt and freshly ground black pepper

6 fresh sage leaves, finely chopped, plus extra for garnish

1 sheet nori, julienned, for garnish

Place the lentils in a large saucepan and cover with 1$\frac{1}{2}$ cups of the broth. Bring to a simmer over medium heat and cook, uncovered, until the lentils are tender, about 25 minutes. Stir in the garlic, sweet potato, celery, onion, tomatoes, and the remaining 2$\frac{1}{2}$ cups of broth. Continue to cook, uncovered, for about 20 minutes, or until the sweet potato is tender. Stir in the miso, kale, and sage. Season to taste with salt and pepper, ladle into bowls, garnish with the nori, and serve.

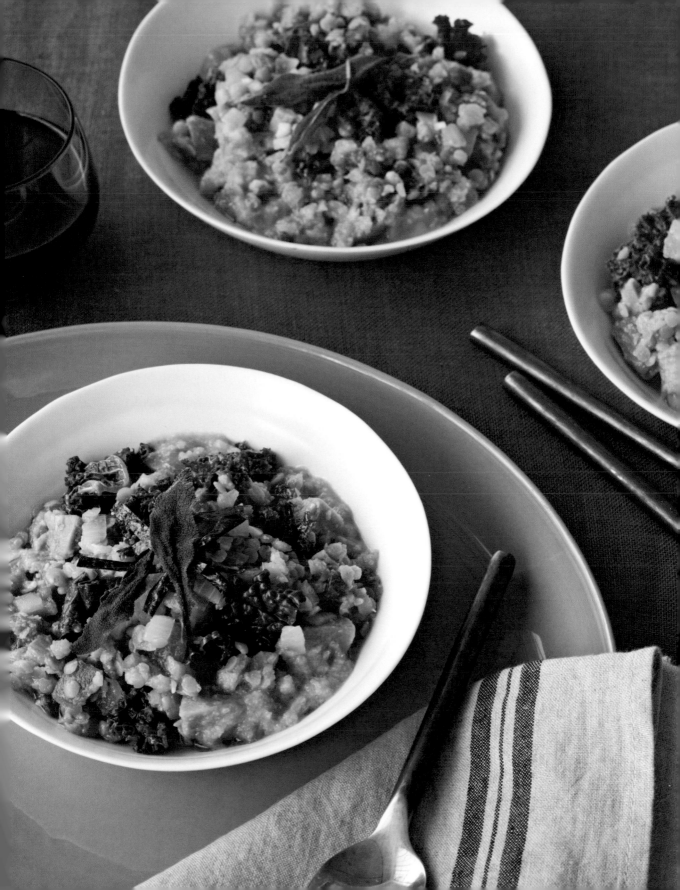

Cannellini Beans with Parsnip and Celery Root

Cannellini beans, which are high in fiber, are the star of this dish. The creamy, buttery legumes are complemented by the sweet earthiness of the root vegetables, but in addition to flavor, the parsnip provides vitamin C and a handful of other vitamins. The herbs and Brain-Boosting Broth supercharge the dish with antioxidants for lots of brain-health support. This dish pairs nicely with a variety of meats—try it alongside lamb or chicken. **MAKES 4 SERVINGS**

2 cups dried cannellini beans, picked over

4 tablespoons extra-virgin olive oil

2 medium parsnips, peeled and diced small

1/2 cup peeled, finely diced celery root

4 tablespoons minced shallot

2 teaspoons dried oregano

2 teaspoons dried thyme

Pinch of ground nutmeg

6 cups Brain-Boosting Broth (page 130)

Salt and freshly ground black pepper

2 tablespoons chopped fresh flat-leaf parsley leaves

Put the beans in a medium bowl and add water to cover by about 2 inches. Let soak at room temperature for at least 6 hours or up to 12 hours. Drain the beans.

In a large saucepan over medium heat, warm the olive oil. Add the parsnips, celery root, shallot, oregano, thyme, and nutmeg and cook, stirring occasionally, for about 3 minutes, or until the vegetables just begin to soften. Add the beans and the broth, increase heat to high, and bring to a boil. Cover; turn down the heat to maintain a simmer; and cook, stirring occasionally, until the beans are tender but not mushy, about 20 minutes. The beans may need an additional 5 to 10 minutes, so check them for doneness. Season to taste with salt and pepper and stir in the parsley. Serve hot.

Condiments and Dressings

Kimchi

In 2009, Beau spent about a month in Korea, where he sampled kimchi, or pickled vegetables, of many different varieties. Kimchi is served at every Korean meal and is known for its vibrant, pungent flavors and aroma and its ability to aid with digestion. Kimchi is rich in vitamins and aids in digestion. This recipe is based on classic napa cabbage kimchi, but the addition of mango and oranges is nontraditional; the fruit adds sweetness that nicely balances the pickles' saltiness and savoriness. Kimchi is commonly used in Korea in stews, soups, and with fried rice. Try serving it alongside Breakfast Fried Rice (page 111). **MAKES ABOUT 3 CUPS**

1 cup coarse sea salt

2 quarts water

2 medium to large heads napa cabbage (about 2^1/$_2$ to 3 pounds each), chopped

1 head garlic, cloves separated, peeled, and trimmed

^{1}/$_2$-inch piece fresh ginger, peeled and chopped

1 tablespoon fish sauce

^{1}/$_2$ cup Korean chile paste (gochujang)

1 tablespoon kosher salt

1 tablespoon sugar

^{1}/$_2$ medium daikon radish (about 6 ounces), peeled and sliced lengthwise into ^{1}/$_2$-inch slices

1 bunch green onions, white and green parts, cut into 1 inch lengths

1 mango, peeled, pitted, and chopped

2 oranges, rinds peeled, sliced into circles

In a large bowl, combine the sea salt and water and stir until the salt dissolves. Submerge the cabbage in the water and let soak at room temperature for 3 to 4 hours.

Combine the garlic, ginger, and fish sauce in a food processor or blender and process until finely minced. Transfer the mixture to a large bowl and add the chile paste, kosher salt, and sugar; stir to combine. Add the daikon and green onions and mix well.

Drain the cabbage in a colander, rinse thoroughly, and drain again. Using your hands, squeeze the heads to remove as much water as possible. Add the cabbage, mango, and oranges to the bowl and mix well, pressing down firmly to remove any air bubbles and making sure all the ingredients are well coated with the seasonings.

Transfer the kimchi to a sealed container. Let stand for 2 to 3 days in the refrigerator before serving. In a sealed container in the refrigerator, the kimchi will keep for up to 2 to 3 days.

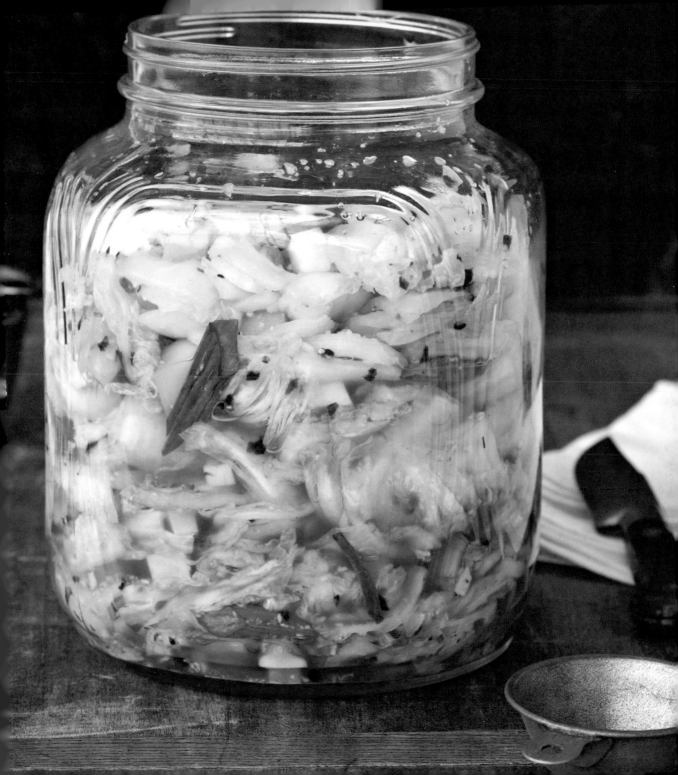

Soy-Sesame Vinaigrette

This is one of the original, best-loved recipes at Beau's restaurant, Elements. When you toss this vinaigrette with some simple mixed greens, it makes a nice, complete salad. The dressing has light notes of soy and ginger, which will appeal to both your senses of taste and smell. MAKES ABOUT 2 CUPS

2 tablespoons peeled, chopped fresh ginger
2 tablespoons chopped garlic
Pinch of red pepper flakes
1/4 cup toasted sesame oil
1/4 cup peanut oil
1/2 cup rice vinegar
1/2 cup mirin
1/2 cup soy sauce
1/2 cup sugar
2 tablespoons cornstarch
2 tablespoons water

Combine the ginger, garlic, red pepper flakes, sesame oil, and peanut oil in a blender and puree until creamy. Pour the mixture into a medium sauté pan and cook, stirring, over low heat until aromatic and golden in color, about 6 minutes.

Add the vinegar, mirin, soy sauce, and sugar to the sauté pan. In a small bowl, combine the cornstarch and water, and then stir the cornstarch slurry into the contents of the pan. Set the pan over low heat and bring the mixture to a boil to thicken, stirring to dissolve the sugar, about 2 minutes.

Transfer the dressing to a bowl and let cool. Cover and refrigerate for up to 1 week.

Mint-Lime Yogurt

Toasted cumin and coriander add spice to this super-simple recipe. It's great served as a dip for crudités, and equally good as a sauce for chicken or fish because its creamy quality adds a delicious richness. Be sure to use low-fat or nonfat yogurt to keep this condiment healthy and low in saturated fat. **MAKES ABOUT 1 CUP**

½ teaspoon ground cumin
½ teaspoon ground coriander
1 cup low-fat or nonfat plain yogurt
2 tablespoons freshly squeezed lime juice
1 tablespoon chopped fresh mint leaves
1 teaspoon grated lime zest
Salt

In a small, dry skillet over low heat, toast the cumin and coriander just until fragrant, a little less than 1 minute.

In a small bowl, mix the yogurt, lime juice, mint, lime zest, and toasted spices. Season to taste with salt. Serve slightly chilled.

Spinach Pesto Yogurt

This Mediterranean-inspired, brain-healthy recipe gets its health benefits from polyphenol-rich spinach and olive oil, and vitamin E is supplied by the pine nuts. Serve this flavorful condiment with grilled or roasted vegetables (it's especially tasty with roasted beets). It's also great as a dressing for a salad of chopped romaine lettuce. Or you can use it as a dip for crudités or toasted pita chips. **MAKES ABOUT 3 CUPS**

2 cups loosely packed baby spinach
1 cup extra-virgin olive oil
¼ cup pine nuts
2 tablespoons grated Parmigiano-Reggiano cheese
1 clove garlic, peeled
Juice of 1 lemon
Pinch of salt
Pinch of freshly ground black pepper
1 cup low-fat or nonfat plain yogurt

Combine the spinach, olive oil, pine nuts, cheese, garlic, lemon juice, salt, and pepper in a blender and puree until well blended. Pour the mixture into a bowl, add the yogurt, and whisk until incorporated. Serve slightly chilled. The mixture will keep in an airtight container in the refrigerator for 3 to 4 days.

Caponata

Caponata is a Sicilian eggplant relish, and it's a dish that is very characteristic of the Mediterranean diet. Many of the ingredients in this recipe support brain health: the vegetables are high in vitamin C and vitamin E, the olive oil and Kalamata olives are great sources of monounsaturated fats, and the anchovies provide omega-3 oils. Caponata may be low in saturated fat, but with so many tasty ingredients, it's got high-impact flavor. Serve it on grilled bread, spoon it on top of hummus for starters, or offer it alongside grilled fish as part of a main dish. You'll find other ways to serve it, to be sure. MAKES ABOUT 2½ CUPS

1 large Italian eggplant (about 12 ounces), cut into ¼-inch cubes

1 teaspoon kosher salt, plus more for seasoning

1 small red bell pepper

5 celery stalks, cut into ¼-inch cubes

5 tablespoons extra-virgin olive oil

1 small onion, chopped

¼ cup red wine vinegar

1½ tablespoons sugar

3 to 4 medium plum tomatoes (about 10 ounces), peeled, seeded, and chopped

¼ cup Kalamata olives, pitted and chopped

1½ tablespoons nonpareil capers, rinsed and chopped

2 oil-packed anchovies, bones discarded and fillets finely chopped

Freshly ground black pepper

In a large bowl, toss the eggplant with 1 teaspoon kosher salt. Let stand for 1 hour; the eggplant will soften and release some of its moisture.

While the eggplant stands, roast the red pepper in the oven at 375°F on a baking sheet, on the grill, or held over a flame on a gas oven with tongs. Char the skin, rotating it for even charring, for 5 to 8 minutes. Once the skin starts cracking, place the pepper in a small bowl and cover the bowl with plastic wrap for 5 minutes. The skin will steep and separate from the pepper so that you can peel it off easily. Once the pepper is cool, peel and seed it, then chop into ¼-inch cubes.

Meanwhile, bring a small saucepan of salted water to a boil over high heat. Add the celery and blanch for less than 1 minute, or until the celery is bright green and softened in texture. Drain, rinse under running cold water, and drain again. Set the celery aside.

Drain the eggplant in a colander and squeeze gently with your hands to remove additional liquid.

In a medium nonstick skillet over medium-high heat, warm 2 tablespoons of the olive oil. Add half of the eggplant and cook, stirring occasionally, until nicely browned. Transfer to a bowl. Repeat with additional olive oil and the remaining eggplant. Season to taste with pepper.

In the same skillet over medium heat, warm the remaining 1 tablespoon of olive oil. Add the onion and cook, stirring occasionally, until tender, about 5 minutes. Add the vinegar and sugar and cook until the vinegar is reduced to a glaze. Add the tomatoes and cook, stirring occasionally, until the moisture evaporates and the mixture is slightly thickened, about 10 minutes.

Add the tomato mixture to the eggplant along with the celery, roasted pepper, olives, capers, and anchovies and mix well. Season to taste with salt and pepper and drizzle in additional olive oil, if desired. Serve at room temperature. This recipe is best served fresh, but it can be kept in an airtight container in the refrigerator for up to 5 days.

Spicy Peanut Sauce

This is a great, flavorful sauce that people really enjoy. It has many different uses—to accompany pot stickers, dumplings, or summer rolls, for example. It's also a very versatile sauce for proteins (especially grilled chicken), sautéed vegetables, or soba noodles. The ginger and chile give this savory sauce just the right amount of spice—Beau prefers sambal chile paste. MAKES 1 CUP

2 teaspoons vegetable oil

2 teaspoons peeled, chopped fresh ginger

2 teaspoons chopped garlic

1 1/2 tablespoons chopped green onions, white and green parts

1/3 cup creamy peanut butter

1 teaspoon Asian chile paste

1 tablespoon rice vinegar

2 tablespoons soy sauce

2/3 cup light coconut milk

Heat the oil in a medium skillet over medium heat. Add the ginger, garlic, and green onions and cook, stirring, until fragrant, about 1 minute, taking care not to brown the garlic. Add the peanut butter and chile paste and whisk until smooth.

Add the rice vinegar, soy sauce, coconut milk, and whisk well. Use right away at room temperature.

Spiced Dried-Fruit Compote

Beau's favorite way to enjoy this easy-to-make compote is over plain steel-cut oatmeal, but it's also terrific as a savory accompaniment, particularly alongside grilled pork or chicken. It keeps well, so it's a handy thing to have on hand. The compote is rich in antioxidants and vitamins thanks to the dried fruits and orange juice. The cinnamon is an additional source of antioxidants. MAKES ABOUT 2 CUPS

1 cup dried figs, quartered

1 cup dried apricots, quartered

1/2 cup dried cranberries

1/2 cup coarsely chopped dried papaya

1 cup water, plus more as needed

1 cup freshly squeezed orange juice

1 tablespoon grated orange zest

1 cinnamon stick

1 star anise

Combine all of the ingredients in a medium saucepan and bring to a boil over high heat. Turn down the heat to maintain a gentle simmer; cover; and cook, stirring occasionally, until the fruits are plump and softened and the liquid has reduced to a syrupy consistency, 35 to 40 minutes. Add additional water if the mixture appears too dry. Transfer to a bowl and let cool. The compote will keep in an airtight container in the refrigerator for up to 1 month.

Applesauce with Ginger and Cinnamon

This ginger-infused applesauce can be served as a condiment or snack, or even as dessert. Made without any sugar except for the natural sugars in the apples and apple juice, it's a healthy way to satisfy a sweet tooth. Cinnamon's warm, spicy flavor and aroma is a natural pairing with apples; the spice is also packed with antioxidants, so you can enjoy this applesauce knowing that you're also supporting brain health. **MAKES ABOUT 1 CUP**

6 Gala apples (about 1^1/$_2$ pounds), peeled, cored, and chopped, 1 cup of skins reserved

1 cinnamon stick

1 tablespoon peeled, minced fresh ginger

2 cups apple juice

1 tablespoon champagne vinegar

Ground cinnamon

Enclose the reserved apple skins and the cinnamon stick in a double thickness of cheesecloth and secure with kitchen twine.

In a medium nonreactive saucepan over medium heat, cook the ginger and apples, stirring occasionally, until the ginger is fragrant and the apples have begin to soften, about 3 minutes. Add the apple juice, vinegar, and apple-skin sachet, increase the heat to medium-high, and bring to a simmer. Turn down the heat to maintain a gentle simmer, and cook until the apples are completely tender, about 1 hour.

Remove and discard the sachet. In a blender, puree the apple mixture until smooth.

Serve warm or at room temperature, sprinkled with ground cinnamon. The applesauce will keep in an airtight container in the refrigerator for up to 4 days.

Resources

ORGANIZATIONS

The Alzheimer's Association

www.alz.org
1-800-272-3900

New fact sheets, informational brochures, and publications are frequently posted on this website, most of which are available as free downloads, and printed copies may be available through local Alzheimer's Association chapters. The website keeps current statistics on Alzheimer's in the United States. The Alzheimer's Association staffs a helpline that is always available. They can provide crisis counseling and can direct callers to resources in the local geographical areas.

Alzheimer's Foundation of America

www.alzfdn.org
1-866-AFA-8484

This organization can provide information about local resources in any geographic area and can provide contacts for social workers.

The American Health Assistance Foundation

www.ahaf.org
1-800-437-2423

The American Health Assistance Foundation provides information about caregiving, prevention, housing, research, and guidance on financial and legal matters.

The Banner Alzheimer's Institute

www.banneralz.org
602-839-6900

This institute has started a National Alzheimer's Registry and the Alzheimer's Prevention Initiative.

The National Institute on Aging (NIA)

www.nia.nih.gov/alzheimers
www.alzeheimers.org
1-800-438-4380

The NIA has an Alzheimer's disease education and referral center. Their site gives important information about diagnosis, treatment, medical breakthroughs, scientific advances, latest conferences, research centers, and clinical trials.

RECOMMENDED READING

Doraiswamy, P. Murali, MD, Lisa P. Gwyther, MSW, with Tina Adler. *The Alzheimer's Action Plan: The Experts' Guide to the Best Diagnosis and Treatment for Memory Problems.* New York: St. Martin's Press, 2008.

Lawlis, Dr. Frank, and Dr Maggie Greenwood-Robinson. *The Brain Power Cookbook: More Than 200 Recipes to Energize Your Thinking, Boost Your Mood, and Sharpen Your Memory.* New York: Plume, 2008.

Maccaro, Janet. *Brain Boosting Foods.* Lake Mary, FL: Siloam Books, 2008.

Peretta, Lorraine, and Oona Van Den Berg. *Brain Food: The Essential Guide to Boosting Brain Power.* New York: Sterling Publishing, 2002.

Sabbagh, Marwan, MD. *The Alzheimer's Answer: Reduce Your Risk and Keep Your Brain Healthy.* Hoboken, NJ: Wiley, 2008.

Shankle, William Rodman, and Daniel G. Amen, MD. *Preventing Alzheimer's: Ways to Help Prevent, Delay, Detect, and Even Halt Alzheimer's Disease and Other Forms of Memory Loss.* New York: Perigee Trade, 2005.

Small, Gary, MD, and Gigi Vorgan. *The Alzheimer's Prevention Program: Keep Your Brain Healthy for the Rest of Your Life.* New York: Workman Publishing Company, Inc., 2011.

Winter, Arthur, MD, and Ruth Winter, MS. *Smart Food: Diet and Nutrition for Maximum Brain Power.* Lincoln, NE: ASJA Press, 2007.

Notes

CHAPTER 1

1. Reynolds, Gretchen, "How Exercise May Keep Alzheimer's at Bay," *New York Times*, January 18, 2012.

CHAPTER 2

1. Paul Zane Pilzer, *The Wellness Revolution* (Hoboken, NJ: Wiley, 2003).

CHAPTER 3

1. M. C. Morris, D. A. Evans, J. L. Bienias, P. A. Scherr, C. C. Tangney, L. E. Hebert, D. A. Bennett, R. S. Wilson, and N. Aggarwal, "Dietary Niacin and the Risk of Incident Alzheimer's Disease and of Cognitive Decline," *Journal of Neurology, Neurosurgery, and Psychiatry* 75, no. 8 (August 2004): 1093–99.

2. In the Baltimore Longitudinal Study of Aging, participants who took folic acid at or above the required daily allowance of 400 mcg daily had a 55 percent reduced risk of developing Alzheimer's. Another study from New York confirmed the protective effects of folic acid consumption. In that study, the group with the highest folic acid intake had a 50 percent risk reduction, compared with the group taking the lowest amount of folic acid. In the study, the highest amount of folic acid was defined as greater than 480 mcg daily. M. M. Corrada, C. H. Kawas, J. Hallfrisch, D. Muller, R. Brookmeyer, "Reduced Risk of Alzheimer's Disease with High Folate Intake: The Baltimore Longitudinal Study of Aging," *Alzheimer's & Dementia: The Journal of the Alzheimer's Association* 1, no. 1: (July 2005): 11–18.

CHAPTER 4

1. C. B. Pocernich, M. L. Bader Lange, R. Sultana, and D. A. Butterfield, "Nutritional Approaches to Modulate Oxidative Stress in Alzheimer's Disease," *Current Alzheimer Research* 8, no. 5 (August 2011): 452–69.

2. D. Benton and G. Roberts, "Effect of Vitamin and Mineral Supplementation on Intelligence of a Sample of Schoolchildren," *The Lancet* 331, no. 8578 (January 1988): 140–43.

3. S. G. Yang, W. Y. Wang, T. J. Ling, Y. Feng, X. T. Du, X. Zhang, X. X. Sun, M. Zhao, D. Xue, Y. Yang, and R. T. Liu, "Alpha-tocopherol Quinone Inhibits Beta-amyloid Aggregation and Cytotoxicity, Disaggregates Preformed Fibrils, and Decreases the Production of Reactive Oxygen Species, NO, and Inflammatory Cytokines," *Neurochemistry International* 57, no. 8 (December 2010): 914–22.

4. Data from the Chicago Health and Aging Project showed that dietary vitamin E was linked to lower rates of cognitive decline, especially among APOE ε4 carriers. The Rotterdam study also suggests that long-term dietary intake of both vitamins C and E has an ameliorative effect on cognitive health, particularly among smokers. M. C. Morris, D. A. Evans, C. C. Tangney, J. L. Bienias, R. S. Wilson, N. T. Aggarwal, and P. A. Scherr, "Relation of the Tocopherol Forms to Incident Alzheimer Disease and to Cognitive Change," *The American Journal of Clinical Nutrition* 81, no. 2 (February 2005): 508–14.

5. USDA Database for the Oxygen Radical Absorbance Capacity (ORAC) of Selected Foods, Release 2. Prepared by Nutrient Data Laboratory, Beltsville (MD) Human Nutrition Research Center (BHNRC), Agricultural Research Service (ARS), US Department of Agriculture (USDA), May 2010 (http://ndb.nal.usda.gov/ndb/foods/list).

6. G. Cao, R. M. Russell, N. Lischner, and R. L. Prior, "Serum Antioxidant Capacity Is Increased by Consumption of Strawberries, Spinach, Red Wine, or Vitamin C in Elderly Women," *Journal of Nutrition* 128, no. 12 (December 1, 1998): 2383–90; G. Cao, S. L Booth, J. A. Sadowski, and R. L Prior, "Increases in Human Plasma Antioxidant Capacity after Consumption of Controlled Diets High in Fruit and Vegetables," *The American Journal of Clinical Nutrition* 68 (1998): 1081–87.

7. C. B. Pocernich, M. L. Bader Lange, R. Sultana, and D. A. Butterfield, "Nutritional Approaches to Modulate Oxidative Stress in Alzheimer's Disease," *Current Alzheimer Research* 8, no. 5 (August 2011): 452–69.

8. J. A Joseph, B. Shukitt-Hale, N. A. Denisova, R. L. Prior, G. Cao, A. Martin, G. Taglialatela, P. C. Bickford, "Long-Term Dietary Strawberry, Spinach, or Vitamin E Supplementation Retards the Onset of Age-Related Neuronal Signal-Transduction and Cognitive Behavioral Deficits," *Journal of Neuroscience* 18, no. 19 (October 1, 1998): 8047–55.

9. M.C. Morris, D. A. Evans, C.C. Tagney, J. L. Bienias, R. S. Wilson, "Associations of Vegetable and Fruit Consumption with Age-Related Cognitive Change," *Neurology* 67, no.8 (October 24, 2006):1370–6.

14. P. P. Zandi, J. C. Anthony, K. M. Hayden, K. Mehta, L. Mayer, and J. C. Breitner, "Cache County Study Investigators—Reduced Incidence of AD with NSAID but not H2 Receptor Antagonists: The Cache County Study," *Neurology* 59, no. 6 (September 24, 2002): 880–86.

15. J. A. Sonnen et al., "Nonsteroidal Anti-Inflammatory Drugs Are Associated with Increased Neuritic Plaques," *Neurology* 75, no. 13 (September 28, 2010): 1203–10.

16. V. Chandra, R. Pandav, H. H. Dodge, J. M. Johnston, S. H. Belle, S. T. DeKosky, and M. Ganguli, "Incidence of Alzheimer's Disease in a Rural Community in India: The Indo-US Study," *Neurology* 57, no. 6 (September 25, 2001): 985–89.

17. J. M. Ringman et al., "A Potential Role of the Curry Spice Curcumin in Alzheimer's Disease," *Current Alzheimer Research* 2, no. 2 (April 2005):131–36.

18. Ann Bartkowski, "Turmeric for Inflammation," www.livestrong.com, May 2, 2010.

19. A. Frydman-Marom et al., "Orally Administered Cinnamon Extract Reduces B-Amyloid Oligomerization and Corrects Cognitive Impairment in Alzheimer's Disease Animal Models," *PLoS One* 6, no. 1 (January 28, 2011): e16564.

20. B. Qin, K. S. Panickar, and R. A. Anderson, "Cinnamon: Potential Role in the Prevention of Insulin Resistance, Metabolic Syndrome, and Type 2 Diabetes," *Journal of Diabetes Sciences and Technology* 4, no. 3 (May 1, 2010): 685–93.

21. Y. J. Wang, P. Thomas, J. H. Zhong, F. F. Bi, S. Kosaraju, A. Pollard, M. Fenech, and X. F. Zhou, "Consumption of Grape Seed Extract Prevents Amyloid-Beta Deposition and Attenuates Inflammation in Brain of an Alzheimer's Disease Mouse," *Neurotoxicity Research* 15, no. 1 (January 2009): 3–14.

22. B. Shukitt-Hale, F. C. Lau, A. N. Carey, R. L. Galli, E. L. Spangler, D. K. Ingram, and J. A. Joseph, "Blueberry Polyphenols Attenuate Kainic Acid-Induced Decrements in Cognition and Alter Inflammatory Gene Expression in Rat Hippocampus," *Nutritional Neuroscience* 11, no. 4 (August 2008): 172–82.

23. B. Shukitt-Hale, F. C. Lau, and J. A. Joseph, "Berry Fruit Supplementation and the Aging Brain," *Journal of Agriculture and Food Chemistry* 56, no. 3 (February 13, 2008): 636–41.

24. F. C. Lau, B. Shukitt-Hale, and J. A. Joseph, "Nutritional Intervention in Brain Aging: Reducing the Effects of Inflammation and Oxidative Stress," *Sub-Cellular Biochemistry* 42 (2007): 299–318.

25. L. Rossi, S. Mazzitelli, M. Arciello, C. R. Capo, and G. Rotilio, "Benefits from Dietary Polyphenols for Brain Aging and Alzheimer's Disease," *Neurochemical Research* 33, no. 12 (December 2008): 2390–400.

CHAPTER 6

1. See the "Know Your Fats" page of the American Heart Association website: www.heart.org/HEARTORG/Conditions/Cholesterol/PreventionTreatmentofHighCholesterol/Know-Your-Fats_UCM_305628_Article.jsp#.TzqhdV0XmjE.

2. S. Kalmijn, L. J. Launer, A. Ott, J. C. Witteman, A. Hofman, and M. M. Breteler, "Dietary Fat Intake and the Risk of Incident Dementia in the Rotterdam Study," *Annals of Neurology* 42, no. 5 (November 1997): 776–82.

3. P. Barberger-Gateau, C. Raffaitin, L. Letenneur, C. Berr, C. Tzourio, J. F. Dartigues, A. Alpérovitch, "Dietary Patterns and Risk of Dementia: The Three-City Cohort Study," *Neurology* 69, no. 20 (November 13, 2007): 1921–30.

4. M. C. Morris et al., "Fish Consumption and Cognitive Decline with Age in a Large Community Study," *Archives of Neurology* 62, no. 12 (December 2005): 1849–53.

5. V. Solfrizzi, F. Panza, V. Frisardi, D. Seripa, G. Logroscino, B. P. Imbimbo, and A. Pilotto, "Diet and Alzheimer's Disease Risk Factors or Prevention: The Current Evidence," *Expert Review of Neurotherapeutics* 11, no. 5 (May 2011): 677–708.

6. K. Yurko-Mauro, "Cognitive and Cardiovascular Benefits of Docosahexaenoic Acid in Aging and Cognitive Decline," *Current Alzheimer Research* 7, no. 3 (May 2010): 190–96.

7. A. D. Dangour et al., "A Randomized Control Trial Investigating the Effect of n-3 Long Chain Polyunsaturated Fatty Acid Supplementation on Cognitive and Retinal Function in Cognitively Healthy Older People: The Older People and n-3 Long Chain Polysaturated Fatty Acids (OPAL) Study Protocol," *Nutrition Journal* 5 (August 31, 2006): 20.

CHAPTER 7

1. N. Scarmeas, Y. Stern, R. Mayeux, and J. A. Luchsinger, "Mediterranean Diet, Alzheimer Disease, and Vascular Mediation," *Archives of Neurology* 63, no. 12 (December 2006): 1709–17.

2. P. Barberger-Gateau, C. Raffaitin, L. Letenneur, C. Berr, C. Tzourio, J. F. Dartigues, and A. Alpérovitch, "Dietary Patterns and Risk of Dementia: The Three-City Cohort Study," *Neurology* 69, no. 20 (November 13, 2007): 1921–30.

3. N. Scarmeas, Y. Stern, R. Mayeux, J. J. Manly, N. Schupf, and J. A. Luchsinger, "Mediterranean Diet and Mild Cognitive Impairment," *Archives of Neurology* 66, no. 2 (February 2009): 216–25; C. Féart, C. Samieri et al., "Adherence to a Mediterranean Diet, Cognitive Decline, and Risk of Dementia," *Journal of the American Medical Association* 302, no. 6 (2009): 638–48; N. Scarmeas et al., "Physical Activity, Diet, and Risk of Alzheimer Disease," *Journal of the American Medical Association* 302, no. 6 (2009): 627–37.

4. P. J. Smith, J. A. Blumenthal, M. A. Babyak, L. Craighead, K. A. Welsh-Bohmer, J. N. Browndyke, T. A. Strauman, and A. Sherwood, "Effects of the Dietary Approaches to Stop Hypertension Diet, Exercise, and Caloric Restriction on Neurocognition in Overweight Adults with High Blood Pressure," *Hypertension* 55, no. 6 (June 2010): 1331–38.

Index

MEASUREMENT CONVERSION CHARTS

VOLUME

U.S.	IMPERIAL	METRIC
1 tablespoon	$1/2$ fl oz	15 ml
2 tablespoons	1 fl oz	30 ml
$1/4$ cup	2 fl oz	60 ml
$1/3$ cup	3 fl oz	90 ml
$1/2$ cup	4 fl oz	120 ml
$2/3$ cup	5 fl oz ($1/4$ pint)	150 ml
$3/4$ cup	6 fl oz	180 ml
1 cup	8 fl oz ($1/3$ pint)	240 ml
$1^1/4$ cups	10 fl oz ($1/2$ pint)	300 ml
2 cups (1 pint)	16 fl oz ($2/3$ pint)	480 ml
$2^1/2$ cups	20 fl oz (1 pint)	600 ml
1 quart	32 fl oz ($1^2/3$ pint)	1 l

TEMPERATURE

FAHRENHEIT	CELSIUS/GAS MARK
250°F	120°C/gas mark $1/2$
275°F	135°C/gas mark 1
300°F	150°C/gas mark 2
325°F	160°C/gas mark 3
350°F	180 or 175°C/gas mark 4
375°F	190°C/gas mark 5
400°F	200°C/gas mark 6
425°F	220°C/gas mark 7
450°F	230°C/gas mark 8
475°F	245°C/gas mark 9
500°F	260°C

LENGTH

INCH	METRIC
$1/4$ inch	6 mm
$1/2$ inch	1.25 cm
$3/4$ inch	2 cm
1 inch	2.5 cm
6 inches ($1/2$ foot)	15 cm
12 inches (1 foot)	30 cm

WEIGHT

U.S./IMPERIAL	METRIC
$1/2$ oz	15 g
1 oz	30 g
2 oz	60 g
$1/4$ lb	115 g
$1/3$ lb	150 g
$1/2$ lb	225 g
$3/4$ lb	350 g
1 lb	450 g